MY BLUEPRINT FOR SUCCESSFUL AGEING

First published in 2025.

National Library of Australia Cataloguing-in-Publication data:
My Blueprint for Successful Ageing / **Gary Shiels**

978-1-7644164-0-5 (paperback)

Cover, illustrations, text design and typesetting: Les Thomas
Editor: Erin O'Dwyer

MY BLUEPRINT FOR SUCCESSFUL AGEING

Live healthier, stronger, longer!

Dr Gary A Shiels AM

Dedicated to my beloved mother who taught me so much about ageing; to our son who taught us the importance of living life; and to my wife who has been my rock and stuck with me through the good and difficult times.

ACKNOWLEDGEMENTS

It is my pleasure to acknowledge and thank the many people who have assisted me during my research and the preparation of this book. I would start with my prime motivator for this book, my late mother for her love and teaching over the time I had with her, and latterly the experience I gained as a carer through her ageing process.

Secondly, I would thank the many people at UNSW who assisted me with my research and PhD. This book draws on my PhD thesis, which was entitled Planning for Successful Ageing in an Age Friendly Built Environment, which was awarded in 2016. Special mention to my key supervisors, Professor Susan Thompson and Dr Peter Williams, who were always there for me.

Thirdly, I would thank the Elders, who invited me into their lives and shared their secrets about healthy longevity. I would also thank the health professionals for sharing their experiences with me on the complex topic of ageing.

Fourthly, I would thank the team at GSA Planning, who supported me through my PhD, with a special thanks to Michelle for her incredible tolerance and input.

Fifthly, I would thank the foreword providers for their very humbling comments, their friendship and support over time.

I would also thank the North Bondi Surf Club, which has been an integral part of my life for the past 60 years; this great voluntary organisation has taught me many of life's lessons.

My penultimate thanks are to my editor Erin O'Dwyer, graphic designer Les Thomas and Tim Castle for their guidance in this process.

Finally, and most importantly, I would acknowledge my life partner and soulmate Vicki, for her ongoing support and sacrifice during the preparation of my PhD and this book. Vicki, thank you so much!

CONTENTS

FOREWORDS

Firstly, may I say what an honour it is to write this foreword to Gary Shiels' book. Gary has had a profound impact on my life – something he may not fully realise until he reads these words.

I first met Gary in the early 1980s when, at 16, I joined the North Bondi Surf Life Saving Club. At the time Gary was club president. I'd been raised by a single mother in a strict Anglican household with my aunt, two sisters, and a brother somewhat older than me who was travelling the world by the time I was seven. So, stepping into the vibrant world of North Bondi Surf Club and finding strong male role models was both unexpected and fortuitous. Gary became one of those role models. He had that rare ability to combine the authority of a president with the camaraderie of 'one of the boys' – a balance I've tried to emulate in my own years as president of the club.

Gary's professional and community contributions are extraordinary. His services to town planning and the community earned him the Member of the Order of Australia (AM) on Australia Day 2023 – a fitting recognition of a lifetime devoted to public good.

Academically, Gary holds three Master's degrees and a PhD focused on successful ageing in an age-friendly built environment. His research spans nutrition, exercise and strategies for healthy ageing. He continues to share this knowledge through presentations, a dedicated website and regular stretch and exercise classes he has run for over 30 years.

A lifetime resident of North Bondi and Managing Director of GSA Planning for 33 years, Gary remains as energetic as ever – coaching, mentoring, swimming and competing. His mission, or *ikigai*, is clear: to help people age successfully.

Gary is an inspiration to many. His enthusiasm for life is infectious, his generosity in sharing research and wisdom unmatched. The pages that follow are a gift: a distillation of decades of knowledge, service and passion.

It is a privilege to introduce this work and to invite you into Gary's world of insight and optimism. May you find, as I have, that his words motivate you to live fully and age well.

Steve Larnach – President, North Bondi Surf Club

At a sprightly 80, Dr Gary Shiels AM distils for us the essence of a lifetime's passionate devotion to maximising healthful longevity both for himself and anyone else who cares to listen. Written by a vastly experienced life coach and significant contributor to his community, this is not a recipe book – it is rather a well-referenced kitchen benchtop workbook requiring self-questioning at various stages along a process of preparing a gourmet meal by utilising only the best ingredients.

It is estimated that at least one third of our societal ill-health trajectory is self-modifiable, and this little book takes us on a veritable tour de force through all the current schools of thought relating to optimal mind and body maintenance, covering such topics as diet, exercise, sleep and attitude.

Discretionary choice and immutable chance are the absolute bipolar determinants of our health trajectory, and by teaching us how to maximise good choice in the face of chance (particularly genetic), Gary enables students to best self-determine their health futures.

On a purely personal note, I believe that it is largely Gary's enthusiastic rehabilitation of my poorly muscled body 20 years ago, which led to me being able to delay the otherwise expected decline in my health due to Parkinson's disease onsetting some 10 years later.

Ted Arnold, MBBS (Syd), MSc(HealthEd) (London), FRACMedAdmin, FACLifestyleMed

I have known Gary for nearly 25 years, through my long-standing involvement with the North Bondi Surf Club – where he is a distinguished 60-year Life Member and Club Patron. Over the years, our paths have also intersected professionally, as well as through shared interests in golf, the gym and the swimming community. I have also attended the fitness class that he runs.

Gary is someone who genuinely lives by the principle 'practice what you preach'. He has always been meticulous about his health, fitness and nutrition, firmly believing that 'you have to look after your body' and 'you are what you eat'. This philosophy is evident in every aspect of his life. Whether it's training and competing at a national level in Masters surf ski and beach running events, swimming regularly in squads, or setting ambitious personal goals, like completing 78 laps of a 50m pool to celebrate his 78th birthday, Gary's commitment is unwavering. His discipline, consistency and drive are nothing short of inspiring.

In keeping with his lifelong dedication to health and wellbeing, Gary undertook a PhD around the age of 60. As part of his thesis, he interviewed 20 older people who were ageing well, and 20 health professionals specialising in ageing. These interviews provided the critical components for successful ageing that Gary seeks to share with everyone in his book.

If there is anyone who exemplifies the knowledge, discipline and mindset required to age not just gracefully, but exceptionally well, it is Dr Gary Shiels. This book provides his blueprint to help all of us to enjoy a healthier, stronger and longer life.

Dr David Digges, BDS, JP, Former NSW Volunteer of the Year

Dr Gary Shiels AM is a born teacher, who cares deeply about you and your wellbeing, and shows you the way by his example. That is the essence of this book. At the heart of Gary's philosophy is a belief that you can control how you age, by commitment to exercise, healthy eating and a positive mindset. All of this can lower your biological age and extend the healthy years of your life. This is what Gary calls your 'health span'.

Gary's blueprint is ideally suited to the 45+ demographic, particularly, but not exclusively, men. In his day-to-day mentoring of myself and others, Gary takes you on a journey to understand the 'what to do', as well as the 'why to do it'. Through this book, Gary offers you and all his readers the benefit of his knowledge and experience, with a personal history to enable you to truly understand what drives him – through both the triumphs and the disappointments of life.

Having been involved in the Wellbeing Committee at the NSW Bar, I can strongly recommend and endorse this book as a call to action for all of us. How we look after ourselves now, also prepares us for the future. I am often reminded of the saying 'when the student is ready the teacher appears'. Take this book, as I have done with Gary's direct mentoring over the last 12 years, as a gift. Some of the advice is tough, and the ideas can be uncompromising. However, Gary will always tell you 'life is not a dress rehearsal'. Best of luck with your own journey and may this book change your perspective on successful ageing.

Tim Castle, B.Ec, LLB, BA (Hons), MBA (Exec)

INTRODUCTION

Growing older in the lucky country

Australia is the greatest country in the world, with the best beaches, highest standard of living, high levels of employment, and one of the best health systems. We have great opportunities for education and the potential to pursue your chosen profession or trade if you are prepared (and have capacity) to work. With superannuation and the potential for various pensions, many older people are encouraged to retire by age 65, and if they have the means, become grey nomads touring Australia or cruising the Mediterranean. Due to financial imperatives, some may need to keep working.

Regardless of our lifestyle life circumstances, when there are opportunities available to enjoy life after 65, why haven't we all learnt how to age well? Ageing well is easier said than done. But it *can* be done. And we can draw inspirations from centenarians and the longest-lived people on this planet and study the attributes of the world's so-called Blue Zones, where Elders are active and productive over their lifetime. The term Blue Zones was coined by explorer Dan Buettner to describe five areas around the world, which have the longest-lived people. They include Okinawa, Japan; Sardinia, Italy; Nicoya, Costa Rica; Ikaria, Greece; and Loma Linda, California. In those places, people were found to be living active, healthy lives into their

90s and beyond. They also have clean arteries, and an absence of some of the health problems found in Western societies.[1]

It's tempting to wonder: if that's where people live the longest, could we all simply pack our bags, move to Okinawa or Sardinia, and become centenarians or even supercentenarians ourselves? Because, regardless of where we live, wouldn't we all like to be able to look forward to being healthy and active when we are 80, 90 and even beyond?

Throughout my career as an urban planner, I have worked on countless seniors housing projects and worked with many providers of aged care facilities. The facilities that promote successful ageing offer residents a healthy lifestyle, physical activity, healthy food, engagement with other residents, and provide the important lifestyle factors that are essential for older people as they age. Some facilities that I have visited are more concerned with the bottom line than offering a healthy lifestyle to their residents. The telltale signs are limited staff numbers, inactivity of residents and poor quality of food. Older people in these facilities seem to sit from dawn until dusk, without being exposed to any movement, stimulation or exercise. They are waiting to die. By comparison in the so-called Blue Zones, centenarians and supercentenarians are climbing stairs, tending gardens and practising tai chi. We live in the greatest country on earth – so why aren't we ageing like it? Why aren't our Elders thriving, instead of sitting silently in the shadows? Do we need to consider a move to the 'enlightened' Blue Zones to age well?

---

1 Blue Zones. https://www.bluezones.com

As part of my PhD research, conducted between 2004 and 2016, I explored the components of successful ageing. I interviewed 20 older Australians (I call them Elders), reviewed the research on the Blue Zones and considered the lifestyle of long-lived people. As part of my earlier research, I also interviewed 20 eminent health professionals, who worked with older people. I was not just considering how we might extend the quantity of life; I was also considering how we might improve the quality of life in our later years. In other words, how can we get our health span to equal, or get close to, our lifespan. Health span is a term used to describe the years that are free from any significant chronic disease or any significant disability that might affect our quality of life. Lifespan, of course, is the length of time a person lives.

In putting together this book, I also visited one of the Blue Zones – Okinawa, and three cities on mainland Japan including Hiroshima, Kyoto and Tokyo – to consider whether it might be somewhere where my wife and I might like to spend more time and thus perhaps extend our lifespan. To visit Okinawa has been a dream of mine since I first read Drs Bradley and Craig Willcox, and Makoto Suzuki's book *The Okinawa Program: How the World's Longest-Lived People Achieve Everlasting Health and How You Can Too* in 2001, and later Dan Buettner's 2008 book *Blue Zones*. I will discuss what I discovered in Okinawa later on in this book. For now, let's just say it strengthened the theory that I put forward in this book – that you can create your own blueprint for successful ageing wherever you live – whether it's Sydney, Sardinia or San Francisco.

An ageing, unhealthy population

Ageing is something we all do while we are taking breath. When we stop breathing, we stop ageing. We all breathe and age differently and the way we age determines the quality of life we will enjoy in our golden years. The figures tell a sobering story. For a nation that prides itself on quality of life, Australia is falling short on ageing well. Life expectancy has increased by around 50% since the 1900s, primarily because of medical advances.[2] At the time of writing this book, the average life expectancy in Australia is 81.1 for males and 85.3 for females. There is also new Australian Bureau of Statistics (ABS) data which records the healthy average life expectancy (known by the acronym HALE), which is approximately 10 years less than the average life expectancy figures.[3] What this means, for the last 10 years of life, the average older Australian is no longer enjoying a healthy life, which concerns me greatly. In many cases this HALE is reduced by 20 years.

First things first: we have a serious weight problem. Australia is ranked 10th out of 21 OECD countries for the proportion of people aged 15 and over who live with overweight or obesity, with the proportion of overweight or obese Australians greater than the OECD average of 59%.[4] Two in three or 66% of Australians are overweight or obese – 34% are overweight and

---

2 AIHW. (2025). *Life expectancy*. https://www.aihw.gov.au/reports/life-expectancy-deaths/deaths-in-australia/contents/life-expectancy

3 ABS. (2025). *Life expectancy*.

4 AIHW. (2024). *Overweight and obesity*. www.aihw.gov.au/reports/overweight-obesity/overweight-and-obesity

32% are obese.[5] Around 63% of men and 72% of women have a risky waist circumference.[6] In addition, almost 1.9 million Australians live with diabetes.[7] Japan, the healthiest country, has 5% of people in the obese category.[8]

Most older Australians spend their bonus years below the disability threshold, which means they need assistance on a regular basis. In 2025, a group of West Australian researchers reported that one in three Australians aged over 70 take five or more different medications.[9] They found that older Australians go to the doctors five times a year, and to the pharmacy 16 times a year. Meanwhile, the number of older Australians using five or more regular PBS medications increased by 32% (from 1.03 million to 1.35 million) from 2013 to 2023, likely driven by population ageing. The simultaneous use of multiple medicines by a patient is known as polypharmacy. Doctors I have interviewed agree that it is not possible to anticipate the side effects from taking multiple forms of medication.

Nor are we moving our bodies enough. The ABS 2022 National Health Survey found that only one in three (33.4%) of people aged over 65 met the physical activity guidelines of

---

5 AIHW. (2024). *Overweight and obesity.*

6 AIHW. (2024). *Overweight and obesity.*

7 Diabetes Australia. *Diabetes in Australia.* www.diabetesaustralia.com.au/about-diabetes/diabetes-in-australia/

8 OECD. (2023). *Health at a glance 2023.* https://www.oecd.org

9 Quek, H.W., Lee, K., Etherton-Beer, C., Lee, G.B., Preen, D.B., Sanfilippo, F., Almeida, O.P., & Page, A.T. (2025). Dispensing patterns of prescription medicines among older Australians from 2013-2023. *Journal of the American Medical Directors Association*, 26(11), 105827. https://doi.org/10.1016/j.jamda.2025.105827 (Quek et al., 2025)

30 minutes or more on most, preferably all, days a week.[10] This exercise benchmark is considered to be better than nothing but is in fact so inadequate as to be laughable. ABS figures reveal that sedentary patterns of behaviour increase with age. Australian Institute of Health and Welfare (AIHW) figures show that around 4.2 million Australians are over 65, around 16% of the population and growing. Around 1.8 million Australians are 75 or over, and half a million are over 80.[11] Some 82% of Australians aged 65+ do not meet physical activity guidelines. Among 65-74 year olds, it is 30%; among 75-84 year olds, it is 23%; and among the 85+ it is 11%.[12] What is hopeful is that, at the other end of the spectrum, 47% of men and 38% of women completed 150 minutes or more of exercise in the last week.[13]

But the stark fact is that three in four Australians aged 65 and over are overweight or obese, with the prevalence increasing with age. In the 65-74 age group, eight in 10 or 78% are overweight or obese, compared with 65% of those aged 18-64 years.[14] In the 75+ age group, 74% of men are overweight or obese, and 65% of women.[15] In the 80-84 cohort some one in five (19%) are living with diabetes – a strong indicator that most people over 80 are sedentary.[16]

10 ABS. (2023). *National Health Survey.* (ABS, 2023).

11 AIHW. (2024). *Older Australians.* https://www.aihw.gov.au/reports/older-people/older-australians/contents/summary

12 AIHW. (2024). *Older Australians.*

13 AIHW. (2024). *Older Australians.*

14 AIHW. (2024). *Older Australians.*

15 AIHW. (2024). *Overweight and obesity.*

16 AIHW. (2024). *Diabetes: Australian facts.* https://www.aihw.gov.au/reports/diabetes/diabetes/contents/summary

It is not our fault that we become sedentary; we are encouraged to do less and take it easy as we age. The problem is that our bodies begin to decline from age 35, if we do not continue to use them. Our muscles, tendons, tissues, joints, cells and brain power atrophy without use, which leaves us susceptible to dementia, cancer and heart disease. Dementia, classified as the progressive decline in people's functioning, is now the leading cause of death in Australia.[17] Obesity, smoking, excessive alcohol consumption, high blood pressure, depression and diabetes all increase the risk of developing dementia. If dementia is now our most serious health threat, the pressing question is: what can we do differently today to prevent it tomorrow?

Move your body

I firmly believe exercise is the closest thing to a panacea for successful ageing. It is also one of the most critical tools in the fight against dementia, and the catalyst which keeps our bodies functioning, repairing and growing. We must continually challenge our heart and lungs – for they enjoy the challenge. Education, good nutrition, cognitive activity, social connection and sleep are also vitally important.

Being sedentary is akin to waiting to die. If we are sedentary, our muscle mass and strength declines, our metabolism slows, and our heart and lung health declines. This can be followed by sarcopenia (loss of muscle mass associated with ageing and immobility), and reduced bone density. If we don't do any exercise over a period of time, our body will think we are commencing

---

17 AIHW. (2025). *Dementia in Australia.* https://www.aihw.gov.au/reports/dementia/dementia-in-aus/contents/about

the dying process and begin shutting down. The less we do, the less we can do. This is not the way we want to spend our twilight years. And ageing doesn't need to be like this! In this book, I will argue that maintaining strength and muscle mass is an important investment for a healthy lifestyle that can increase your health span and make your last years on this planet much more enjoyable.

A graceful way to age

To understand ageing well, we need to start with the limits of human life itself. The maximum life potential (MLP) is the age of the longest-lived member of our species. Researchers argue it is something that cannot be extended.[18] Frenchwoman Jeanne Calment holds this record currently. When she died at age 122 years and 165 days, she was reportedly in good health, though almost blind and deaf.[19] While healthy long-lived people are uncommon in Western society, the Elders I interviewed are an exception. They live or lived in Australia, mainly NSW, where they have created their own blueprint for successful ageing.

I will discuss these long-lived people in Chapters 3, 4, 5 and 10, but here is a brief intro to the Elders I became aware of or met during my research:

> **Catherina van der Linden** passed away on Australia Day 2024 in South Australia at age 111. She credited her longevity to her active lifestyle.

18 See, for example, Fries, J. & Crapo, L. (1981). *Vitality and ageing*. WH Freeman & Co.

19 Australian Institute of Health and Welfare. (2025). Dementia in Australia. https://www.aihw.gov.au/reports/dementia/dementia-in-aus/contents/about

Ken Weeks is Australia's oldest living person. He is 111 and lives in an aged care facility in Grafton in northern NSW. He attributes hard work, baked beans and a happy life for his longevity.

Dr Gladys McGarey was a remarkable 103-year-old North American, who passed away in September 2024, and was referred to as the mother of holistic medicine. She had many recommendations for healthy longevity, including exercise, and limiting the quantity (and improving the quality of) food.

Peter Manner, who died in 2025 aged 101 is one of my role models. I was fortunate enough to attend Peter's 100th birthday celebration at the Wine and Food Society of NSW. Right up until his death, he swam, kept active, had a purpose in life, and enjoyed a tipple of red wine.

Not everyone can be a centenarian or a supercentenarian, but the closer I get towards that age myself, the more I think it is not beyond our grasp.

In this book, I will endeavour to convince you it is your biological age, which is important, not your chronological age; and I am going to help you to lower your biological age. I am grateful for the experiences I have had in life, and I am pleased to have the opportunity to give back. Hopefully, I will be able to help you!

Many of us would like to think we can age well and be swimming, running, walking, gyming, dancing or playing golf well into our 80s, 90s and beyond. While this is distinctly possible, a paradigm shift will most likely be needed. Each of the Elders I interviewed had identified the components that were critical for them to enjoy a long and healthy life, and they had created those components in their living environment. No matter what your age is, if you want to do any, or all, of the above activities as you get older, you need to start preparing for it now. And remember, you don't get old, you get older!

In the following sections, I am going to set out my blueprint for successful ageing. It has three parts to it: a strategy, a paradigm, and a selection of three age curves. First is my 'A-List Strategy', which has five separate yet related elements, that I would ask you to adopt as your mantra for living life. Secondly, I am asking you to adopt my Successful Ageing Paradigm – which may well involve a paradigm shift, if indeed you want to become a healthy, long-lived person. A paradigm is a set of concepts, based on research, and is a distinct way of looking at life. A paradigm shift is a fundamental change in approach or underlying assumptions. In other words, I am encouraging you to change your mindset and discard the misinformation all of us have been fed throughout our lives and adopt the A-List Strategy and Successful Ageing Paradigm I have set out in this book. You can then select one of the three ageing curves, which will complete your blueprint for how you will age.

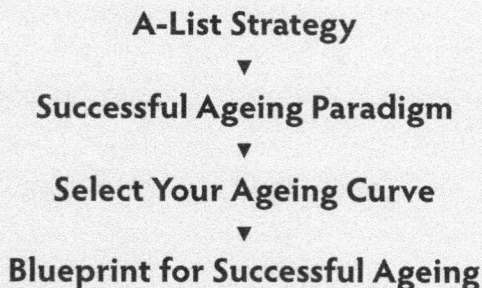

A-List Strategy
▼
Successful Ageing Paradigm
▼
Select Your Ageing Curve
▼
Blueprint for Successful Ageing

A-List Strategy for successful ageing

I have used established research and research from my PhD to formulate my blueprint for ageing successfully. Firstly, let me explain my A-List Strategy. Remember at school, being told to try to get 'As' and stay away from 'Ds'. Well, nothing has changed. We still want to be at the top of the class! However, you don't necessarily have to be the smartest kid in the class (I never was) or have the highest IQ. You just need to be able to adopt these simple strategies as your mantra for life and you will be an A-grader. Adopting the five 'As' – attitude, activity, adventure, appreciation and associations – is the foundation of your blueprint for ageing successfully.

> **Attitude** – A positive attitude is the most important characteristic you can have as you approach life. It gives you the confidence to pursue anything – most importantly, in the context of ageing, exercise and a healthy lifestyle. A positive attitude provides you with the *chutzpah* to get out of bed in the morning and go training. Additionally, extensive research by Dr Becca Levy, PhD, the lead researcher of a study conducted at Yale University's Department of Epidemiology and Public Health, found that a positive attitude adds a further 7.5 years to your life expectancy.[20]

> **Activity** – This is something you should pursue every day for as long (and as strong) as you can. There are many activities you can pursue, and I will discuss most of these in the following pages. Activity is essential for successful

---

20 Levy, Becca, PhD. https://becca-levy.com

ageing. I consider activity to be anything that moves mind, body or limbs. There is considerable discussion in this book about activity, or exercise as I prefer to call it, and Chapter 1 and 7 deal with the topic in some detail.

Adventure – This should be a critical part of life. Explore new options, look for new challenges and enjoy different things. There is nothing better to raise the heart rate than being in a race, being on a wave or skiing down a slope. It could also be a walk in nature or a swim in the ocean or river. Anything where you are on the edge of being in, or out of, control. The adrenaline rush helps keep you young.

Appreciation – We should appreciate our Elders and long-lived people for their wisdom and lived experiences. They can teach us how to age well. We should also express gratitude every day that we are alive and well in this amazing country.

Associations – Our relationships should be retained, nurtured and developed throughout life. Having strong associations with family, friends, sporting buddies, volunteer organisations and our church, is important for our wellbeing. Avoid the naysayers and negative people, they will not help you on your quest for healthy longevity.

In contrast to the five 'As', I urge you to avoid the five 'Ds'. These are decline, disability, decrepitude, disease and dependency. By avoiding them, we can break the stereotypical ageing model. Focus on the 'As', rather than the 'Ds', and do your best to enjoy the hell out of every day!

Successful Ageing Paradigm

My Successful Ageing Paradigm embraces my A-List. However, now I am asking you to adopt the healthy ageing research and discard the popular belief that you should do less as you age. I want you to believe you can do more – and enjoy it more.

My Successful Ageing Paradigm is not a fairytale and is based on numerous case studies and research literature. However, as I will remind you throughout this book: *If you think you can, or if you think you can't, you are probably right!* The critical elements of my Successful Ageing Paradigm are as follows:

- Your chronological age is irrelevant. It is your biological age which is important, and you can lower your biological age – 60 is your new 40; 80 is your new 60; and 100 is your new 80.
- The five 'As' – attitude, activity, adventure, appreciation and associations – are your new mantra for life.
- The five 'Ds' – decline, disability, decrepitude, disease and dependency – are not mandatory or inevitable (and can be deferred or avoided).
- You are now an A-grader, not a D-grader in this world – and you have the confidence, drive and commitment that goes with it to decide on your ageing curve.
- Establish your short-, medium- and long-term goals, then prepare your own personal exercise program (PEP) to help you achieve those goals. I will discuss this further in Chapter 7.

Going forward I encourage you to enjoy each moment, as it is precious. Keep these two catchphrases in mind:

- *Carpe diem* – 'seize the day' in Latin – enjoy the pleasures of the moment without dwelling on the past or being overly concerned about the future.
- *Ichi-go ichi-e* is a Japanese four-character idiom (*yojijukugo*) that describes a cultural concept of treasuring the unrepeatable nature of a moment. Many miss the pleasures of the now, worrying about the past or future.

Also, as I will remind you throughout this book, remember: *Life is not a dress rehearsal!*

If you can adopt these strategies as your mantra for life, and embrace the successful ageing paradigm, you are then well placed to select your successful ageing curve, where most of you can enjoy a greater quality of life into your 80s, 90s or even as a centenarian. Having adopted your blueprint for ageing successfully you can determine your goals and the program to achieve them, wherever you live.

You have probably met 80-year-olds who look like they are 60 and thought: *I wish I could be that fit, at that age.* Well, the good news is, you can. A long-term friend of mine, John, recently turned 80. To celebrate he swam two laps of Bondi Beach (approximately 2km) with a few friends. Halfway along they stopped and sang Happy Birthday. His son gave him a T-shirt (which he now proudly wears), which reads, *It took 80 years to look this good!*

The overarching change I am asking you to make is to take responsibility for the way you age and the way you live your life. Some of you already do this – at least partly or maybe even fully. Those who don't, stop blaming your parents for your genes or any health issues that you think are holding you back from pursuing exercise and a healthy lifestyle. We all have genetic legacies and many of us have injuries – from playing football, basketball, skiing or whatever, either in early or later life.

Many of my friends who were incredibly fit when they were younger suffered an injury at some point and stopped exercising. Some have gained 10 or 20kg, which is life-threatening. My mission is to help you to get fit, and keep you fit, so you can have a healthy and fulfilling life – and age well. We need to stop using genetics and injuries as an excuse not to exercise. Instead, we have to overcome and work around them. If you have a problem, work out how it can be resolved. If you are not active, have a medical check-up before starting exercise, to ensure you do not have any underlying health problems. Don't accept advice from anyone who says that it is okay to do nothing and be sedentary. Exercise is not negotiable. It is a critical part of successful ageing.

Exercise is one of the most important factors in healthy ageing. Exercise can change mindsets, cure depression, prevent cancer, and keep your heart and lungs healthy. The good news is that exercise does not need to cost you anything. In fact, it can save you a lot of money, with less trips to the doctor and a lot less medication. Don't rely on the medical profession to get you fit and keep you healthy; they are geared to fix you up when you become unwell. When was the last time your GP prescribed exercise? If they did, hang on to them, they are rare in my experience. The medical profession and the pharmaceutical companies (Big Pharma) make their money treating unwell or injured patients. It is in their best financial interests for you to be unhealthy.

Another important factor is diet or nutrition. Nutrition fuels the body and allows it to function and pursue exercise and other activities. High quality nutrition allows your body to perform at a high standard and avoid disease. However, as I will introduce in this section and discuss in Chapter 9, we live in a world of deception. We should be able to rely on product packaging when it says it is healthy; however, most of it is at best disingenuous and at worst dishonest. How can a sugary drink in a 375ml can, with 8-12 teaspoons of sugar be described as healthy? Similarly, how can refined food with additives recognised as carcinogens be described as good for you?

The debate about whether exercise or diet is most important in our health and wellbeing is an old one. There were once two gentlemen who had contrasting views on whether exercise was enough in isolation, or whether it needs to be accompanied by a healthy diet. The first was James Fixx, who argued that it didn't matter what you ate if you did plenty of exercise. Hamburgers and fast food were high on his menu. Fixx dropped dead during a marathon, after suffering a massive heart attack due to three blocked arteries. In contrast, one of my role models, the late US fitness trainer Jack LaLanne, recognised the importance of a good diet and a properly structured exercise routine. LaLanne's mantra was 'Exercise is King, Nutrition is Queen, put them together and you have your Kingdom'. LaLanne lived an exceptional life, which changed the way we think about exercise today. I'll talk more about LaLanne later in this book.[21]

Although exercise is almost a panacea for successful ageing, and nutrition is an essential companion, there are many other factors that will determine whether you age well. Sleep, social support and avoiding addictions are other factors, and will be discussed later in this book.

Select your ageing curve

In my PhD research, I developed a series of ageing curves which I believe provide a powerful visual blueprint for understanding how lifestyle choices impact the rate and quality of our physical and cognitive decline as we age. My work stood on the shoulders of Dr Ralph Paffenbarger, Stanford professor, ultramarathon runner, pioneer in the field of physical activity epidemiology, and author of *LifeFit*, which set out a guide for lengthening and improving lives.

Dr Paffenbarger maintained that 'it is never too late to take up an active life' and became so convinced by his research that at age 45 he took up jogging. In his early 80s, he had more than 150 marathons and ultramarathons to his credit. The ageing curves I have included in these pages are built on earlier work by Paffenbarger and Olsen, which I have modified in my research.[22]

21 Britannica. *Jack LaLanne*. https://www.britannica.com/biography/Jack-LaLanne
22 Paffenbarger, R. & Olsen, E. (1996). *LifeFit*. Human Kinetics. (Paffenbarger & Olsen, 1996).

In broad terms, each ageing curve represents your rate of mental and physical decline from age 35 until the ultimate sign-off (death). Sadly, we are all in decline from age 35 and the more risk factors you are exposed to, the faster you will decline. I will discuss risk factors in Chapters 2 and 9. I will briefly discuss these ageing curves now, and in more detail later. There are three ageing curves for you to select from. The one you select will determine how you age.

The first curve is the **usual or typical curve**, which is a steep decline from age 35, broadly representing a ski slope. The majority of our population are pursuing this curve. That is why it is called the usual or typical curve. People on this trajectory are usually sedentary and likely to be overweight or obese. They are likely to require medication, fall below the disability threshold, and require assistance at a younger age.

The second curve is the **optimistic curve**, where there is a lesser decline and a more optimistic approach to lifestyle. Those pursuing this curve are conscious about exercise and lifestyle, although not totally committed to avoiding life's risk factors. Their decline is less rapid than the usual ageing curve and they are likely to spend less time below the disability threshold.

The third curve, the **successful ageing curve**, is for people committed to avoiding the lifestyle risk factors. These people are pursuing regular vigorous exercise and consuming a healthy diet. This curve is theoretically rectangularised, such that people on this curve decline very slowly from age 35, until near to the end, when they drop off the cliff of life. This curve also has the benefit of compressed morbidity and minimising time spent on medication and below the disability threshold. I will discuss these curves, the disability threshold, and the medication zone, in more detail in Chapter 3.

The **successful ageing curve** is our mission. The aim is to get as close as possible to a rectangular ageing curve, which has a high level of wellbeing, is disease-free, and health span equals lifespan. Health span equals lifespan when a person maintains full physical, cognitive and emotional function throughout their entire life, with minimal illness or disability until the very end. This is not just theory; there are real-life examples. We can live healthier, stronger, and longer!

The 20 Elders I interviewed as part of my research lived in the metropolitan areas of Sydney and South-East Queensland and were aged between 80 and 104. They were selected because they were all healthy and ageing well. These Elders had been able to avoid the lifestyle risk factors, which I will discuss later, and pursue a **successful ageing curve**. Some Elders were still working, some were doing voluntary work, and some were pursuing various interests. Importantly, all of the Elders were exercising regularly (if not daily), eating a healthy diet, sleeping well, and they had retained their various social networks.

When I commenced these interviews about 20 years ago, I thought 80 was the beginning of serious ageing, and at that time 80 exceeded the life expectancy for males in this country. What I have discovered, now that I am there, is that your chronological age is irrelevant. It is your biological age which is important. And it is possible to lower your biological age.

In our society, we are continually tempted by lethargy, apathy and misinformation. Comfortable lounges and highly refined foods are promoted as healthy, and seniors are told to take pills rather than exercise. I have a theory on vested interests – that is, that we live in a world of control, power and deception. Most of the stakeholders and interest groups (the culprits), that could help to improve our lifestyle as we age, are driven by their own agendas. The seven culprits in my theory on vested interests are summarised below and discussed in more detail later:

1. **Food manufacturers** that simply want us to eat more, whether it is healthy or not.
2. **Supermarkets** that sell us more than we need, with no regard for health or nutrition.
3. **Medical professionals** who are trained to respond when we are unwell, rather than keep us well. What hope do we have when their mantra is, *do no harm.*
4. **Pharmaceutical companies** that make more money when we are unwell.
5. **The media** that promote any food, alcohol and gambling for financial gain without any moral compass.
6. **Social media influencers** – the mega providers of mis-information – who also receive money for their endorsements, regardless of the truth.
7. **Governments** that don't want to change anything as they are making too much money in taxes and don't want to upset the other co-conspirators.

I'll discuss my theory on vested interests in more detail in Chapter 9.

What we do know is that health outcomes are shaped by external factors as much as internal ones. Life expectancy is reduced for people living with social disadvantage and intergenerational adversity. It's not enough for these people to start eating well and exercising. We need public health policies to address this – to improve health inequities via funding, to make healthy food as affordable as fast food, and to educate people about the dangers of smoking, poor diet and to encourage lifestyle changes. People need to know that no matter what their income or health status, there is support available to improve their health. Almost all of us can improve our health, strength and longevity.

Accordingly, it will take an effort from all of us to bring about change and swing the health pendulum from cure to prevention. If only government took the time to calculate the savings to the national purse from moving to a health prevention model, the national health and greater wellness benefits would be overwhelming. In the meantime, small changes can lead to larger reforms. We need a bottom-up approach, and that starts with all of us.

Why I wrote this book

So, if this is obvious, *why do we need this book*? That is a good question. There are many other books you can read about healthy ageing, and I have read most of them. While some have a similar message, my book is based on academic research and 80 years of experience.

Firstly, with a modicum of bias, I believe my book is compelling, because it adopts the KISS (or Keep It Simple, Stupid) principle, and is based on my real-life experiences and observations. I have documented my daily activities, exercise programs and health issues for the past 60 years, so I have a reasonably good idea of what works for me and what doesn't. I am also doing a few things right – my biological age is closer to 60 than 80; I am not taking any medication; my blood pressure hovers around 115/67; I have the grip strength of a fit 40-year-old; and I exercise for one to two hours every day.

Also, they say you learn by your mistakes, and I have made plenty of those. In my 80th year I set myself two short-, two medium- and two long-term goals, then designed my PEP to meet those goals. I simply wanted to show that age is no barrier, and you are only limited by your own self-belief. I will discuss my goals in the following chapters. Secondly, my research has identified some amazing facts, that I have endeavoured to present in plain English language and largely free of complex medical jargon. Thirdly, my book contains a simple blueprint that can change your life, offer you a healthy ageing trajectory, and a health span that almost equals your lifespan. You won't need to rely on numerous pills or vitamins, and I do not recommend gene therapy.

The other question I am regularly asked is, ***what was your motivation for this book***? Again, a good question. The motivation for this book came from three separate yet related areas in my life.

Motivation One: This came from caring for my mother through the ageing process until she passed away at 96.

She was an amazing lady, who remained positive until the end. There are a few luminaries who passed away at age 96. Her Majesty Queen Elizabeth II lived to 96 – and regardless of whether you are a republican or a monarchist you have to admit she was a very impressive woman. Also, my role model, Jack LaLanne, the father of gymnasiums in the US, and the first person to encourage women to use weights, also passed away at 96.

Motivation Two: I wanted to publish some of the research I could not include in my PhD. In fact, one of my examiners wanted me to delete half of my research and change the topic of my thesis after nine years of study. He kept asking, 'What does a town planner know about health and ageing?' Fortunately, my second examiner thought the topic had considerable merit and was very timely with an ageing population. When I was almost ready to accede to the request by this difficult examiner, to delete the interviews with Elders, one of my supervisors replied, 'Over my dead body'. With the support of my supervisors, we convinced the Higher Degree Committee that the topic and research were timely and that a humble town planner could make a worthwhile contribution in the area of health and ageing.

Motivation Three: This came from a compelling desire to explore and understand why some people are struggling at 60, while others are healthy at 100. Some people in their 60s cannot get out of a chair and wouldn't think of going for a walk or to the gym, while some centenarians are still working from dawn to dusk, go dancing, or are breaking sporting records. I wondered whether it was the luck of the gene pool, was it where people lived, or was it their lifestyle. Should I be moving to the Blue Zones if I want to live to 100 or longer? I also wanted to explore my theory on vested interests, that is that we are continually misled by groups with something to gain, that take us along the path that leads to an unhealthy lifestyle (**usual or typical curve)**, instead of towards a **successful ageing curve**.

In the following chapters, I will endeavour to convince you that it is worth the effort pursuing a healthy lifestyle. Not only will you feel better each day, but you will potentially avoid most forms of cancer and cardiovascular disease. You may find the following chapters confronting, or not to your liking and choose to dismiss this book as being in the too-hard basket. Those of you that persevere to the final chapter will have the information to make an important lifestyle decision – namely how you age. Wouldn't you like to choose the successful ageing curve rather than the usual or typical one? Wouldn't you like the last decade of your life to be full of fun, friends and activity? If so, read on, as I take you on a journey to your new blueprint for successful ageing. Summaries of each of the chapters are included below.

In **Chapter 1**, I will discuss my early family life, growing up in Bondi as a sickly child, who developed a passion for exercise and lifelong learning, and a need to understand what makes our bodies function. I will also discuss the influence that my wife, my mother, the surf club and personal events played in me becoming committed to helping people understand the benefits from a lifelong pursuit of exercise.

The focus of **Chapter 2** shifts to the human body with the strong message that, you have to look after your body, it is the only place you have to live. We will explore our transformation from Neanderthals to Homo sapiens, and the complexity and functioning of the body. We will briefly consider our changing demographic profile, our national health issues, and the risk factors we are exposed to daily. Finally, I will ask you to review the three ageing curves and determine where you are now and where you would like to be moving forward.

In **Chapter 3** we journey to the Blue Zones – communities where people regularly live to 100 and beyond. Their diet and lifestyle hold lessons for all of us. We briefly consider the Okinawan Study, the China Study, and the 20 extraordinary Elders, aged 80 to 104, who were part of my PhD research and embody the blueprint for ageing successfully.

Chapter 4 considers why a positive attitude is one of the greatest attributes you can have to age successfully. This chapter explores how we can develop the habit of being positive, and looks at the secrets of centenarians and supercentenarians, and how their achievements might assist us on the road to positivity. The research informs us that a positive attitude can provide an improved quality of life and an increased lifespan.

Chapter 5 asks you to consider how positive is your attitude. After recapping on some of the positive attributes, the issues with a negative attitude are discussed and the impact that naysayers and stereotyping has on older people. Importantly in this chapter you are asked to undertake a quick quiz to determine, prima facie, which of the three ageing curves best fits your lifestyle.

Chapter 6 deals with nutrition, a critical part of successful ageing. Our historic dietary habits are considered, and several diets are reviewed, from my perspective. The chapter provides Australia's dietary guidelines, and the food and beverages we should be avoiding. I also present my nutritional rules, my preferred foods and my current diet, which is based on my 80 years on this planet. There is also some discussion on food intolerances, the need to avoid unhealthy processed food and the benefits of a Mediterranean diet.

Chapter 7 considers the importance of exercise in our daily routine. After a discussion about the history and the guidelines, the various types of exercise are discussed, and options are provided for you to consider. I present my arguments for vigorous exercise and the need to maintain muscle mass and strength as you age. Finally, I present my approach of establishing goals and developing a personal exercise program to achieve those goals.

Chapter 8 considers the importance of rehabbing the body. Firstly, on a nightly basis when we sleep, and then when we are injured. I also provide some brief discussion about the importance of the spine and ensuring that our lifestyle does not induce back pain. I recount some of the injuries I have had to rehab, then conclude with a short story I wrote, after an emotional journey, my last rodeo.

Chapter 9 deals with addictions, risk factors and vested interests. This chapter asks the question whether there can be healthy addictions and whether the unhealthy addictions make us vulnerable to behavioural or biomedical risk factors. My theory of a world of deception is also discussed and I ask whether there is a conspiracy to keep us unhealthy.

Chapter 10 reviews the components of successful ageing that were identified by the Elders. The chapter reviews how the Elders embraced positive attitude, exercise, sleep nutrition and social connections on a daily basis. Importantly, they all had a purpose for getting out of bed in the morning and all but one had avoided behavioural and biomedical risk factors. The chapter explores how they created their own blueprint for successful ageing.

Chapter 11 presents my final thoughts, the lessons I have learnt during my lifetime and my closing pitch to change your life. The afterword is a reflection on my recent trip to Okinawa, one of the original Blue Zones. I compare the observations first made by Wilcox, Wilcox and Suzuki in 2002, and more recently by Dan Buettner in 2008, and what my wife Vicki and I observed in June 2025. You'll have to read on to learn move, but suffice to say: there's no place like home.

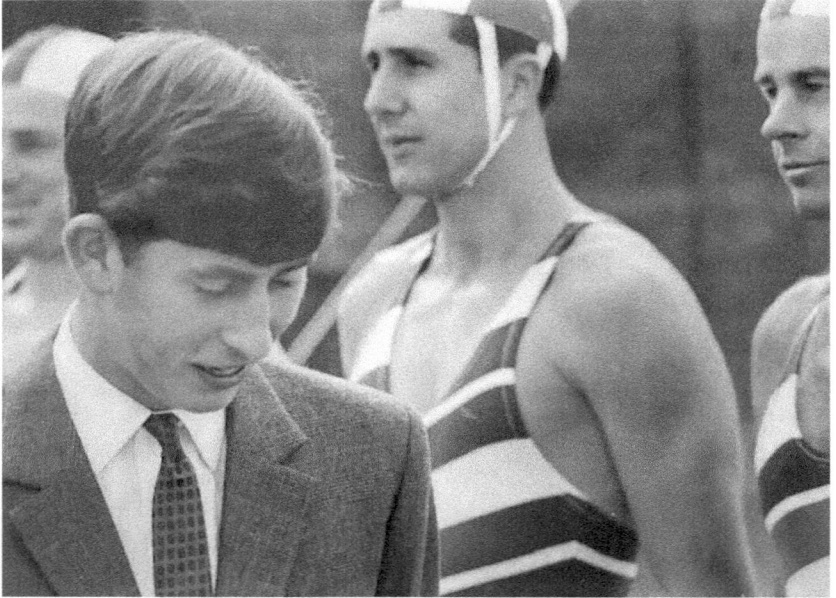

In 1966 the author was fortunate to meet the then Prince Charles when he visited the North Bondi Surf Club. (Gary pictured in the middle of the photo.)

CHAPTER 1: DEVELOPING A PASSION FOR EXERCISE

In the beginning

I was born in the War Memorial Hospital in Waverley in the eastern suburbs of Sydney in December 1945 and lived in a semi-detached dwelling in Blair Street, North Bondi. We had two Pomeranian dogs – Cheeky and Tiny. My mother, Esma Amelia Shiels, who was positivity personified, owned and worked in a small greengrocer shop six days a week, 200m from where we lived. She sold the business shortly after I was born. She then worked as a shop assistant at the Coles department store in the city for many years. Mum was very active in her younger years, and an exceptional swimmer. I always remember her as someone who did not stop moving. For her, there was always something to do. Both Mum and Dad worked just to make ends meet and she would always tell me how lucky we were.

I loved our semi in North Bondi (in fact I have lived my whole life in Bondi). It was 200m from the sewer outlet, otherwise known as 'the stink pipe'. I used to tell people it was a monument. The stink pipe, at the top of Blair Street, became an increasing environmental problem at Bondi Beach. At peak times, raw sewage would be pumped into the ocean without any treatment. Many years later, after intense community pressure, the government would undertake considerable works to upgrade the outlet to provide primary treatment with a deepwater ocean outfall about 1km out to sea.

As a child I was quite sickly, with an inordinate number of food allergies. These included cow's milk, eggs, various forms of dairy and, importantly, the lifesaving drug at that time, penicillin. I also suffered from bronchitis, and being allergic to penicillin, before the days of antibiotics, it was difficult to treat chest infections. If I had a chest infection, I would be confined to bed for long periods of time. There was no medication available for the doctor to use. In later years, my parents told me that there was more than one occasion when they thought I might not recover from a serious bout of bronchitis. Our family doctor affectionately called me his 'problem child'. I grew out of my vulnerability to bronchitis and all my other allergies, except penicillin. I am sure surfing after school and other childhood exercise helped to strengthen my lungs and reduce my susceptibility to bronchitis. Now by choice, I avoid dairy, pork, salt, sugar and by necessity any food containing gluten. As I will explain in a subsequent chapter, I have become gluten intolerant. Also, my current level of exercise is the only medication I take, although I do take a few vitamin supplements.

1950s

In the 1950s, I didn't really know what exercise was and didn't think much about it. Mum and Dad didn't do any exercise, and there wasn't any real encouragement for me to get involved. Although I regularly went to Bondi Beach and rode a surfer plane (a popular pump-up rubber mat in the '50s and '60s),

I couldn't really swim. As Mum swam a lot when she was young, she insisted that I learn and took me to swimming lessons at Alf Vockler's swimming enclosure at nearby Watsons Bay, on Sydney Harbour. Alf was cunningly funny; he would always make statements at the beginning of each swim season that he had never seen so many sharks in Sydney Harbour. It was his covert attempt to encourage swimmers to use his enclosure and pay the entry fee. Mum literally dragged me to Watsons Bay Baths after an unfortunate experience at Bondi Baths, when I was six and my first swim coach physically threw me in the deep end of the pool and said, 'swim'. I never went back to him, and that experience stayed with me until I had several lessons at Watsons Bay. Although I didn't realise it at the time, swimming, surfing and walking to school amounted to a considerable amount of exercise on a daily basis during my school years.

My father was old school and believed that you should never get into debt. When I was seven, our rented semi came up for sale. Rather than pay the £10 deposit required to purchase it, my father moved us into a small flat in the same street (Blair Street), where we again paid rent. When I asked why we were moving, my father replied, 'You never get into debt!' The total cost of our semi was £1000. ABS data would indicate the cost of our semi was about 2.5 times the average annual wage: currently the medium house price in the area is about 13 times the average annual wage.

Houses in Bondi were incredibly cheap in the '50s and '60s compared to today. The smart money was buying houses with some enthusiasm. But my father was immoveable. I was devastated that we had been forced to move out of our beloved semi into a tiny one-bedroom flat where I was sleeping on the veranda. It was then I made my first lifestyle decision – I would never pay rent, and I never have. (Little did I know that once I married, I would move to a third dwelling in the same street – the first semi I purchased with my wife Vicki – and so I was destined to spend the first 40 years of my life living in Blair Street.)

My family's one-bedroom flat was approximately 1.5km to the north of our semi, near an intersection informally known as 'seven ways'. This informal name reflected the convoluted street pattern, where cars and buses converged on a busy seven-lane intersection, adjacent to our flat. Although we were a similar distance from the beach (approximately 2km), it seemed much further. As we lived in a tiny flat with no backyard, we would play in the streets after school – running, climbing and doing all the mischievous things that kids do growing up. At the time, developers were building the Rex Hotel behind the flats where we lived. We would climb the barbed wire fence, have lime fights in the lime pit and have a different adventure each day, not appreciating that we were pursuing dangerous and vigorous exercise. When dark fell, we would return home, assuring our parents that we hadn't been playing in the building site.

I walked to school at Bondi Beach Public, which was about 1km from where we then lived. My report cards would regularly say, 'Gary has considerable potential if he applied himself'. High school was 5km from home, so I would walk part of the way and then get the famous Bondi Tram, which could move more people more efficiently than any other form of transport. The tram fare was one penny and sometimes, when my school mates and I didn't have the fare, or even when we did, we would skulk around the running board on the outside of the tram, to avoid paying the conductor. I think it's fair to say I didn't really apply myself to my studies, although I never really failed anything. At high school the only subject where I showed any potential was technical drawing, and I topped the year. On reflection, this was the first indication I had any aptitude for design and spaces. At school, I was not much of a fan of sport or exercise except surfing.

Both my parents smoked. Dad would have 40 cigarettes a day and Mum would have one or two. I hated the smell of smoke and ashtrays, which resulted in my second major lifestyle decision, that I would never smoke. Dad gave up smoking at 40, but his lungs were shot, and he endured many years of ill-health, before passing away at 85 from the underlying cause, emphysema. Mum and Dad also enjoyed a drink, and Dad would go to the pub every night for a few drinks with his mates. Mum would stay home and prepare the dinner.

1960s

In the 1960s I became hooked on surfing. I had a 10-foot Malibu board, and I would go surfing whenever possible at South Bondi. There were some fascinating characters that were part of the surfing fraternity in those days. Some of those characters included Big Bruce, a man mountain, who loved a fight and wore small men's T-shirts to look even bigger; Rob

Conneeley, a super surfer who won numerous surfing titles; and Bob Barrett, a tough guy who worked on the door at the local night club. Bob would always greet you with the saying, 'You wouldn't be dead for quids!' He went on to write a series of novels about a tough Aussie bloke, Les Norton, who was a mixture of characters including Doogza Davis, a renowned waterfront worker, and himself. Les Norton ended up being a mini-series on TV and is available on Audible. I listened to one of Bob's books recently, entitled *You Wouldn't Be Dead for Quids,* and although it is an acquired taste, I could not stop laughing.

On weekends, a group of South Bondi grommets (young surfers including myself) would go off surfing, in someone's car, whoever was old enough to hold a licence, and we could be anywhere between Crescent Head on the Mid-North Coast of NSW to Tathra on the Far South Coast. We would surf till exhausted, then eat and sleep, normally on the beach. I could write a separate book about the characters at South Bondi at that time, and the famous Astra Hotel potato pies, which were our treat after surfing.

I left school at 14 and got a job at the Department of Motor Transport as a clerk. Money was tight in our household, and it was not uncommon for young people to leave school at that age. My father always said, 'You need to work for the government as you will have job security'. I was not suited to repetitive clerical work however, and I was totally bored. I got my driving permit at 16 and 10 months, and my licence at 17, which were the minimum age for both.

While teaching me to drive, my father always insisted, 'You must drive with five car spaces in front and five car spaces behind at all times, to see other drivers braking or not braking'. I still follow that safety protocol. My father was one of eight children, and he became the breadwinner at age 14, when he and the family left my grandfather in Cooma and moved to Darlinghurst in Sydney. Dad had lived through the Depression and World War II, when money didn't come easily. Accordingly, he was conservative when it came to any expenditure or holidays, which was frustrating for both Mum and me.

Dad was a spare parts salesman for Holden, and he could remember the number of every part, for every car, which normally comprised seven numerals. He had an incredible memory for detail. He also enjoyed the claim to fame of having driven the first Holden cab (taxi) in Sydney. It followed that my first car was a second-hand 48-215 Holden, which became known as the FX, after it was launched by the Prime Minister of the day, Ben Chifley, in 1948. The FX was the first car wholly built in Australia by General Motors Holden, and it was followed by the then-famous FJ Holden (1953-56), which was a similar shape and a little more refined. There was a lot of national pride when Australia got its first, homegrown motor vehicle. It was described as economical, sturdy and stylish and was immediately popular. My Holden seemed to have more room than my veranda space in our flat and I enjoyed driving it everywhere.

My first real trip was to Coolangatta in Queensland to go surfing, with a couple of mates, when I turned 17. I was also playing football with Bondi United, a local rugby league club, and I was selected to play for Eastern Suburbs in the Presidents Cup in 1966. We were beaten by South Sydney that year in the Grand Final. I have been a Roosters (Eastern Suburbs) tragic ever since. The following year I was encouraged to move to rugby union, also playing with Eastern Suburbs. I learnt much about exercise and training, playing both league and union, and recovery after a game on the weekend.

The dynamics of Bondi changed with the increase in car ownership in the '60s. The government had pulled up the tram tracks and taken the trams out of service to make way for cars and buses. I could never understand this decision, and I was too young to understand the politics. Tram tracks became building sites, parks, and parking lots. Our 'cousins' in Melbourne were much smarter and kept their trams, and they are still extremely efficient in that city today. In Sydney, the government is now putting back light rail, where trams once were. Many younger people, who don't know the history of trams in Sydney, comment to me what a good idea it is to be installing light rail!

In 1965, the Prime Minister Harold Holt and his government introduced national service and there was a ballot to decide who would be called up for service and deployed to Vietnam. My name was drawn out in the ballot, and I stupidly embraced the idea at the time. As I was allergic to penicillin, after two medical examinations and an 18 month deferment, the doctors didn't know what to do with me. They couldn't decide whether to enlist me or knock me back as medically unfit. I was frustrated by the bureaucratic indecision, and at the same time I was disenchanted with my job. A mate of mine and I decided to leave work and go to Queensland, a totally irrational decision.

I was working as a barman at South Molle Island, in Queensland's Whitsunday Islands, on the graveyard shift, which started at 1am and finished at 10am, when my mother forwarded me a notice that I was going to be called up. I had to return to Sydney and present myself for another medical examination. This was one of the most outrageous periods in my life. I was going to parties and then going to work; sleep was a non-priority. A group of mates from Bronte arrived at the resort with a one-metre crocodile and it was running around biting people, so I had to resolve the problem. There are many stories from that time that cannot be recounted here. There was no thought of exercise or healthy eating, life was one big party. It would be an understatement to say that I did get into a modicum of trouble, but it would also be an understatement to say I did have a serious amount of fun. Having to return to Sydney and face the music was a reality check, and the first turning point in my life!

Starting to study

On my return from Queensland, I managed to get re-instated at the Department of Motor Transport. They were sympathetic to me returning, as I actually had a reasonable track record, despite my boredom. I also worked part-time at a leagues club as a waiter to save some money to buy a house. (I was still determined I was never going to pay rent.) Other part-time jobs included cleaning industrial oil tanks on weekends, and doing a milk run. My enthusiasm to serve in Vietnam had waned, with reports of injuries and casualties. Also, my mind had moved to a different place. I wanted to learn stuff and be involved in work I enjoyed and be productive.

I heard that there was a road design section in the Department of Motor Transport, and I made enquiries about how I might get involved. My first and second approaches to that section were declined, and I was told I had to complete the Land and Engineering Survey Drafting (L+ESD) Certificate. However, when I tried to enrol, I was told I had to complete my Higher School Certificate (HSC) first. I subsequently enrolled in the HSC at Sydney Technical College at night and completed it in 12 months. This proved to be a major struggle as math had moved on dramatically – it had become calculus and integration, which was a different world to anything I had seen. However, with some tuition, I managed to scrape through my HSC, and in parallel I was enrolled in the first year of the L+ESD Certificate, which I enjoyed.

I kept applying to the road design section and eventually, after about 12 months, they felt sorry for me and gave me a start. This was the second turning point in my life. I was doing work I enjoyed, working in a great team and learning new things every day.

The L+ESD Certificate was an incredibly diverse, four-year course, which addressed everything from sewer and road design to surveying and subdivision. In today's world it would be a diploma or degree. A few colleagues enrolled in a two-year extension course – engineering surveying – so I followed their lead. I thought I was heading towards being an engineer, and had enrolled in an engineering degree, but the only problem there was math, which is important for engineering and not my strong suit. I had somehow managed to pass Math for Surveyors, but not without a lot of work and some help. In the second year of the engineering surveying certificate, I took an elective subject that would change my life yet again. The subject was Town and Country Planning, and the teacher was charismatic. It took me only a few lectures to decide what I wanted to do with my career – I wanted to be a town planner.

In the 1960s, town planning was just being recognised as a profession, and chief engineers were parachuted into chief planner positions and given an honorary Town + Country Planning Certificate. Mere mortals had to go to university and obtain a degree or pass the Town + Country Planners Certificate examinations (known as Ordinance 4).

I started applying for jobs as an assistant town planner at numerous councils and attempted to enrol in a planning degree at various universities. After several knockbacks, I got offered a position as an engineering surveyor/town planner at Ku-ring-gai Council and enrolment at Macquarie University. I grabbed both of these opportunities with great enthusiasm. I am still friends with the chief planner at the council at that time, Charles, who gave me that employment opportunity over 50 years ago. The first year at university was particularly difficult and I almost didn't make the cut. As someone who had left school at 14, I had to lift my standard to a different level academically.

However, Macquarie University got me rolling on what would become an academic snowball. I finished my degree in

Urban Studies, and I was offered enrolment in a new Master's degree that was starting, resulting in a total of seven years of part-time study at Macquarie. I then completed two subsequent Master's degrees – one in engineering science at the University of NSW (UNSW) and another in Urban Design at the University of Sydney. Finally, I completed my PhD, again at UNSW.

As I keep saying, I am a slow learner! However, I had developed a passion for lifelong learning. As all of my studies were part-time, I missed a lot of the university culture that full-time students enjoyed. In contrast, I was working both a full and part-time job throughout. I also became involved in the town planning professional body, The Royal Australian Planning Institute, which then became the Planning Institute of Australia (PIA). I held the position of Councillor then President, at state, national, and international level. For my contribution I was made an Honorary Life Fellow of PIA in 2006.

In 1964, I joined the North Bondi Surf Life Saving Club (North Bondi Club), which gave me an appreciation of exercise and training. Although I was still riding my Malibu board, that was fun, not training. The prerequisite for joining a surf club at that time was swimming 400m in under eight minutes, then completion of a surf lifesaving Bronze Medallion.

The Bronze Medallion involved about 8-10 weeks' training to learn resuscitation and how to perform various rescues. Passing the Bronze meant you were a proficient lifesaver and could undertake voluntary patrols on weekends during the summer months. To remain a proficient lifesaver, you need to renew and refresh your skills annually. I recall, at that time, if you could complete the above, run two laps of the beach and perform 50 sit ups, you were considered to be really fit. I have now been a member of the North Bondi Club for 60 years and I am so grateful to have made so many friends and had so many great experiences.

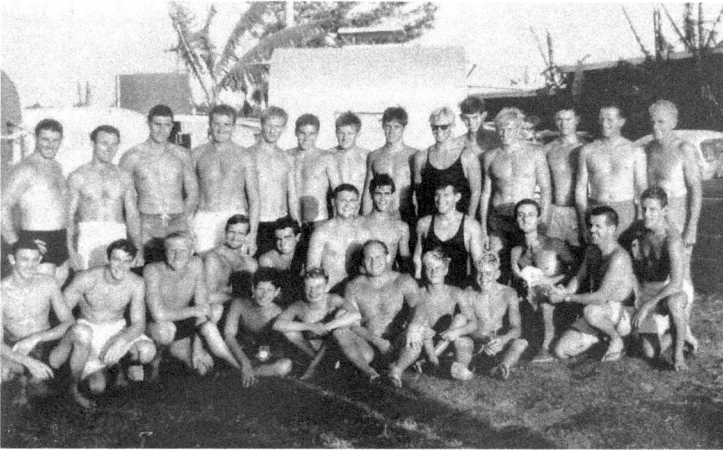

The North Bondi team to the Australian Championships in 1966, held at Coolangatta.

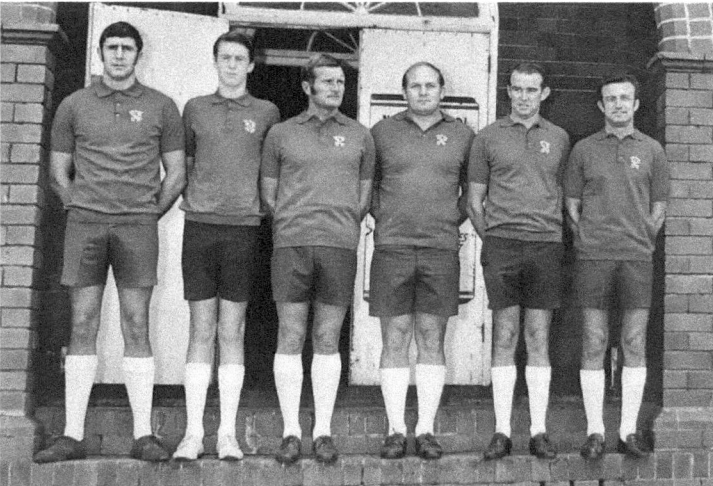

The North Bondi team to the Australian Championships in 1971, in Perth, WA.

13

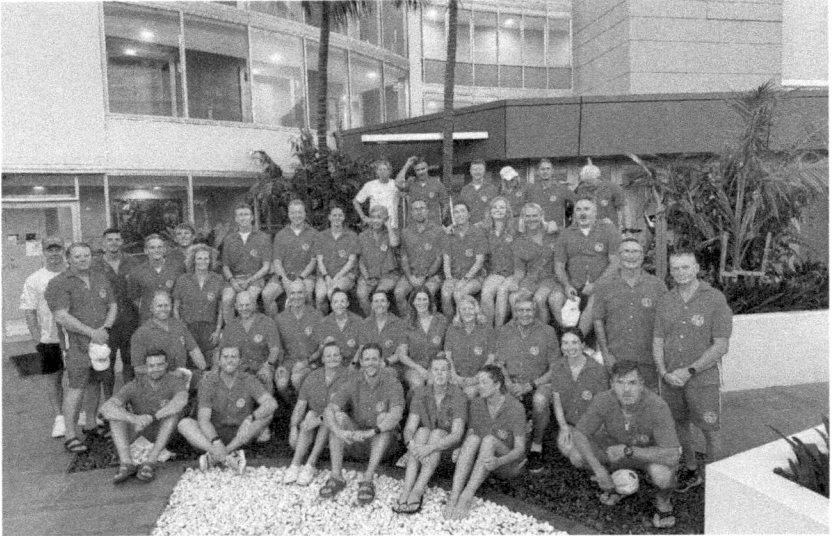

The North Bondi team to the Australian Championships in 2025, in Kirra, Qld.

Ski paddling became the next exercise passion, and we were fortunate enough to win the NSW surf ski teams in 1977, and we were runners up in 1976 and 78. I am still close friends with both Johns, and we regularly come together for a catch-up.

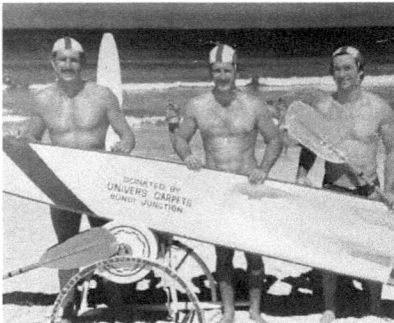

John, John and Gary 1977.

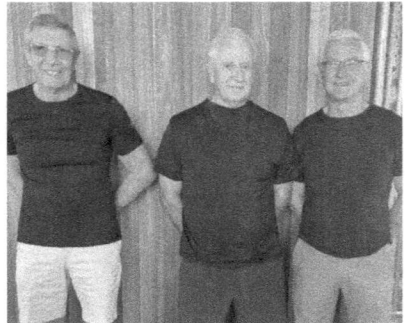

John, John and Gary 2024.

Surf clubs are a great conclave for exercise and for finding role models you can look to for inspiration and guidance. I have been lucky enough to have access to great mentors, who have passed on their wisdom. One of my earlier mentors was Lance Frost, who was like a second father to me, and was always doing work around the club. When I asked him why he was so committed, he replied, 'It was great camaraderie and when you mix with younger people, you stay young'. I have held the positions of Captain, President, Secretary and Public Officer, and was made a Life Member of the club in 1985, and I am currently Club Patron. One of the reasons for this book is to try and pass forward some of those experiences.

1970s running

In the '70s, I discovered running. With the guidance of George Daldry, a world-renowned coach and trainer, I would run 10km, 15km, half marathons and then marathons. George would have his students piggybacking each other up stairs, which was the beginning of back problems for many of us.

We established a committed group of runners who would meet at 5.30am three mornings a week at the Oxford Street Gates in Centennial Park and run either a 10km or 15km course in the park and adjoining green spaces. This was not just a run; it was a great social outing.

In 1971, the first City to Surf was held – a 14km fun run from the Sydney CBD to Bondi Beach. That first year, about 3000 people ran and approximately 100,000 watched. By 2025, it was the reverse – with close to 90,000 running and about 3000 watching. Now known as the City2Surf, it was addictive, with participants trying to better their time each successive year. It has become one of the most popular fun runs in the world and our early Centennial Park runs became part of our training for this annual race.

My first serious City2Surf objective was to break 60 minutes. In the ensuing years, as our training became more intense, I broke 60 minutes and got a preferred start. (A preferred start meant I was allocated space at the front of the pack when the gun went off.) In the late '80s and early '90s, I trained for the City2Surf with well-known ironmen including Guy Leach, Grant Kenny, Scott Thomson, Miles Blackwall, Craig Riddington and Trevor Hendy. Scott and Guy were natural runners with efficient and effortless styles. Craig, with his thick-set frame, struggled and had to work at it. Most people avoid the things they don't like or are not good at. Craig, being a true champion, made running his number one challenge.

These training sessions were always competitive. We trained under Mick Porra, a multi-World and Australian Malibu and Long Board Champion. Under Mick, our training program became much more sophisticated than an ordinary park run. A session might include: a 3km warm-up, 14x400m in 1.15-1.20 minutes and repeating efforts on the 2.00 minutes, finishing with a 3km warm down. That year, which was 1989, most of us ran sub-55 minutes and I recall thinking perhaps I could break the elusive 50 minutes. Craig Riddington ran his personal best and a sub-55. Breaking the 50-minute barrier was the Holy Grail of the City2Surf, given that the fastest-ever time set by

Steve Moneghetti was 40.03 in 1991. Moneghetti's time still stands as the race record.

I ran a total of 33 City2Surfs, a dozen half marathons, numerous triathlons and two marathons. My best time at the City2Surf was 51 minutes, in 1991. I only stopped running when my 'knee vet' said he thought it was time to stop serious running on the concrete. If I kept running on hard surfaces, he said, I would need knee surgery. He said I could keep jogging or walking the event, but somehow that didn't appeal. Now, 35 years on, I am back running, this time on the soft sand.

Endurance events

I have always admired those athletes who compete in ultramarathons. It requires a different level of commitment, an excessive amount of training and a high degree of insanity. In 1982 I trained for the PYE surf ski ultramarathon from Forster to Bondi, only to be struck down with pneumonia one week before the start of the event. As it was a biennial event, I had to wait until 1984 to pursue my goal to complete the event. I was so committed to completing that event that I was training in pitch darkness in the middle of winter at 3.30am three days a week and on weekends with a close friend, Bob Irwin. The other days we did weights.

We were also joined at training by an inexperienced paddler I will call Dr Pete. Racing surf skis are not easy to balance, and as I have always said to beginners, the first five years are the hardest. Dr Pete had only been paddling three months, and he spent a lot of time in the water. That winter was particularly harsh, with freezing cold westerly winds almost every day and a high rain fall level. I recall thinking on several occasions paddling in the dark with 15km westerly winds that I would hate to fall into these icy waters. Dr Pete was doing this regularly. A typical Sunday paddle was four to six hours from Bondi to Manly and return, or Rose Bay to Palm Beach. Our group objective was fundraising for our favourite charities.

The event, which was 270km from Forster to Bondi, was completed over four days and there was a total of 70 starters. The bedraggled group that finished that event was richer for the experience. Notwithstanding the pain, the joy (or relief) of finishing was indescribable. I lost 10kg, had tendonitis in both wrists, no skin on my hands, and sea ulcers on my butt. We had paddled over packs of sharks, experienced 30-50km/h headwinds, suffered hypothermia, and had a near-death experience while lost at sea. Although it was the greatest test ever to my mental and physical endurance, it still rates as the silliest thing I have ever done.

Dr Pete greeted me at the finish line with these words: 'Nothing you do after this will seem difficult.' He was right. That ultramarathon event taught me a great deal about the body's capacity to keep going, even when you think you are physically and mentally spent. It is a lesson that has helped throughout life.

I was fortunate to be Race Director for the first Cole Classic, which was a 1km and 2km swim, held at Bondi in 1983. A few years later, we started running the East Rough Water Swim, which was sponsored by East Rugby Leagues club, when I was again Race Director. These events gave me the opportunity to observe first-hand how older people benefit immensely from this type of activity. Some older people would train all year for both events. These races were their medium- and long-term goals. Some want to win their age group, others just want to complete the course. I was also Race Director for the Foster Sydney Ironman Championship. The objectives of this event were much different. Instead of a safe and enjoyable community event, the emphasis was to provide a spectacular race to showcase these elite athletes for a television audience. While I learnt an enormous amount about exercise from organising these events, it would be my next role that would present the most amazing experience and challenge.

Between 1989 and 1992, I was Race Director for the first three years of the Uncle Toby's Super Series. The series comprised six elite Ironman events, over different distances in four states in Australia, plus one event overseas. The first event was the Gold Coast Gold marathon, a ski paddle, from Surfers Paradise to Coolangatta, then running, swimming and board paddling, back to Surfers – a total distance of 47km.

I was lucky enough to have the support of an incredible team: Dr Bill Roney, a Hawaiian Ironman age group winner; engineer Peter Head; Peter Moscatt, a champion football player; and John Stevens, the In-shore Rescue Boat (IRB) Co-ordinator. This event involved coordinating 40 competitors, 12 surf clubs, and over 200 surf lifesaving volunteers for a four-hour live television event. As the series was live to TV, there were no retakes. The conclusion of this first marathon event was terrifying and heart-stopping. Leaving aside the countless problems we incurred during the race, with five minutes to go before the cross to the 6pm news, it was pitch black, and we had no competitors in sight. Then the helicopter spotlight focused on Guy Leach, who was running along the beach, stretching out towards the finish line. It was great television!

The amount of preparation that these elite athletes were pursuing was phenomenal. They each had what I call personal exercise programs (PEPs), to meet their goals to win races. Their structured training sessions each day embraced swim, ski, board, running and gym. This was their normal routine, and they had one rest day a week.

Two of the Ironmen, Clint Robinson and Grant Kenny, were also training to paddle kayaks at the Olympics and their training workload was slanted towards paddling. Clint Robinson, at age 20, won the first gold medal for Australia ever in the kayaks, winning the K1 1000 in 1992 in Barcelona. I have also had the good fortune of observing the commitment of other Olympians in my surf club, including sprint

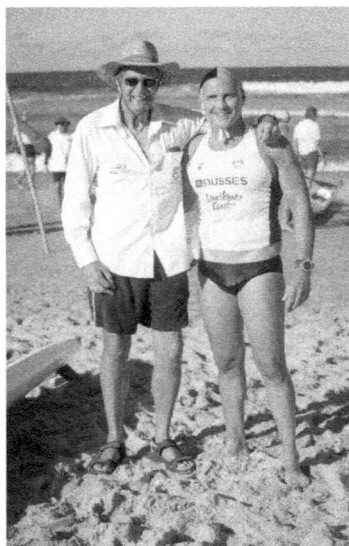

Reunion with Grant Kenny at the Australian Championships in 2024, in Mooloolaba, Qld.

canoeist Jim Walker who competed in the 1996 Atlanta Summer Olympics, and Noah Havard, who won a silver medal in the K4 500m in the 2024 Paris Olympic Games.

Jim Walker, at 50, is still very competitive in open surf ski races and regularly beats guys 25 years his junior. In the lead-up to his Olympic event, Noah Havard advised me he was training six to eight hours a day, six days a week. A typical day might be 30-minute warm-up, two hours paddling (morning and afternoon), abs, 10x10 chin-ups, Pilates, stretching, weights, a massage, a sleep and plenty of food. Havard was consuming an omnivore diet and said it was like throwing logs into a furnace trying to refuel his body from his exercise program. If you put this in perspective, Havard was exercising as much in one day as I do in one week, and I am a dedicated trainer.

I've learnt so much watching Olympians and Ironmen train. Their application, preparation and commitment enabled them to perform at an exceptionally high level, beyond what most of us can even imagine. But what inspires me most is that the same mindset – applied consistently – can help all of us live healthier, stronger, longer lives.

Family life

Vicki and I met in the Rex Hotel in Bondi in 1966. I saw an apparition across the room, with long black hair down to her waist, and I just had to talk to her. She had recently moved to Tamarama from the country, and I was totally besotted. However, our initial relationship was short-lived as I was driving to Perth, in my then EH Holden (manufactured 1963-1965) the following day with a few mates. On my return we dated for about six years before we married in 1972. We would enjoy the beach, going running together and doing active things.

It was an amazing wedding day with surf lifesavers forming a guard of honour at St Marys Church in Bondi, and a horse and carriage to transport us to the reception. I knew nothing about this arrangement, which was organised by one of my groomsmen. The reception was at Bondi Icebergs club, and it was a memorable night.

As Vicki and I were both determined not to pay rent, we were looking for somewhere to buy in Bondi. We eventually found a semi that we both loved, and could almost afford, still in Blair Street. To pay for this overcommitment to purchase our semi I worked two jobs, and we almost never went out. Every dollar we earned went towards paying off our mortgage. Although I didn't have the conservative views of my father of never being in debt, we did want to reduce and eliminate our mortgage as soon as possible. As we mainly had home-cooked meals and few takeaways, our diet was very nutritious. However, fitting in work, family, exercise and study was a constant challenge. Programming study and training in the very early mornings seemed to work reasonably well and we both developed that habit.

We were blessed with a son, and we decided to get another dog, this time a Doberman. We chose a Doberman because they need plenty of exercise. Vicki and I would take Brit with us when we went running. Sadly, Brit passed away from parvovirus and was followed by Pepper, another Doberman, who was an accident looking for somewhere to happen. She would jump off cliffs and got run over by a bus and still survived. She died of a heart attack, walking with Vicki in Centennial Park. Finally, we got Jana, our loveable Border Collie, who captured all of our hearts and controlled everyone with her charm.

Our son, Ryan, was an absolute joy, and we all enjoyed each other's company. Vicki, Ryan, Jana and I would regularly exercise together, with walks and runs along the Bondi Promenade or in Centennial Park. Ryan was incredibly smart and was managing a computer business, in Blair Street at age 15, when his boss was overseas. At age 17, he was taller than me, about 1.84m, lean and hungry, and he had just rejoined the surf club, to my great delight, after a period of absence, and was going into Year 12 at Cranbrook School.

On Australia Day in 1994, we were having lunch with friends when we received a phone call every parent dreads. Ryan had been involved in a serious car accident and was being airlifted to hospital. We leapt into the car. The Air Rescue Service intercepted my car radio and told us the helicopter was going to Westmead Hospital. Then they called back and told us to drive to Royal North Shore Hospital, which is where they decided would be the best venue to treat him.

When we arrived at Royal North Shore Hospital, we were told that he had been driving on a dirt road and rolled the car. He suffered devastating head injuries and was badly brain damaged. I hope no-one reading this has to go through an experience like that. It devastated Vicki and myself. Ryan was on life support for 12 days and we received different opinions as to whether he would survive, and if he did survive, whether he would be in a vegetative state.

I can't begin to tell you how terrible this period in our life was. We were both traumatised and it was not possible to think straight. After 12 days, he contracted pneumonia, and on medical advice, we made the very difficult decision to turn off his life support. Every day, I still wonder whether we made the right decision, or if we could have done something to ensure that the accident didn't happen in the first place. It is true what they say that you never get over the loss of a child. However, if you are going to survive, you have to learn how to live with it.

I remember that I started exercising fanatically. I thought that this would block out the pain and momentarily it did. Exercise was my rabbit hole where I could hide. However, the memories would come rushing back as soon as the physical pain and endorphins from the exercise subsided. Nonetheless, I found that exercise was a great stress reliever, and it did help me to retain a modicum of sanity. Apart from the feeling there was a massive hole in my chest, greeting people was a real problem, for them as much as me. Some days I could talk about it, other days I would burst into tears. Friends would not know what to say, so they would avoid us. We are not really taught to grieve, and when we are thrust into the unthinkable, we are forced to deal with it as best we can. If you know someone who is grieving, it doesn't matter what you say but say something.

Around that time a friend of mine also lost his son, and he decided he could not cope and ended his life. I did have those thoughts on occasion. Somehow, we both managed to overcome the pain. There is not a day that goes by where I don't think about Ryan, and I'm grateful for the 17 years we did have together. I consider myself the luckiest person in the world to be married to such a wonderful person as Vicki, who has supported me for the past 60 years and tolerated my shortcomings. Without a doubt, exercise helped me through this terrible ordeal.

My mother

Mum and Dad had moved to a holiday cottage, on St Huberts Island near Woy Woy, that was accessible only by boat, when they could no longer afford to pay rent in Bondi. Mum had purchased a small fibro dwelling on the island, and the vendor allowed her to pay it off over two years. You cannot do that type of financial arrangement today!

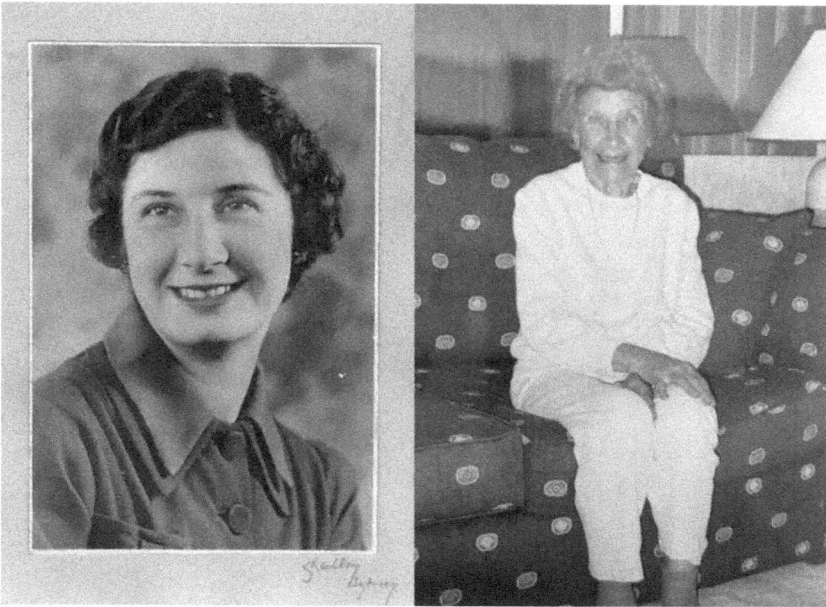

Mum at ages 26 and 86.

Subsequently, a bridge was built to the island, when developers tried to realise the potential, but it was still relatively inaccessible.

Vicki and I would visit Mum and Dad every couple of weeks to help with shopping and maintenance. Dad was unwell for about 15 years, the many years of smoking and lack of exercise taking its toll. He became very frail in his later years and seldom left their little house on the island. When he passed away, at 85, Mum lived on the island on her own, and my trips became weekly, when I would visit and replenish her fridge. We had a surprise 90th birthday party for Mum on the island. I was terrified the surprise party might kill her, but she just took it in her stride, and everyone had a ball. Mum remained on the island until she could no longer manage, and I moved her to a seniors housing unit near us in Bondi.

On moving my dear old Mum from the Central Coast to Bondi, my role as a carer intensified from part-time to full-time. Vicki would also assist with Mum's care. My first task was to review her medication. Although I'm not a medical doctor, I have researched the impacts of long-term use of various forms of medication. Also, my interviews with Elders and health professionals provided some real-life case studies on the optimal use of medication.

Mum was taking 12 different types of medication prescribed by at least three different doctors, which immediately raised my concern whether all of these drugs were necessary. This was beyond polypharmacy! Accordingly, I organised an appointment with a GP, who specialised in older patients. That GP reduced the number of prescribed medications from 12 to four. Before then, no one else had reviewed the whole package. It was a turning point in Mum's care – and a stark reminder of how vital it is to have good holistic care in your older years.

Mum's progression through the ageing process was one of the key motivations for my research. Even at 94 when she was almost blind, her attitude was amazingly positive. She would say: 'If only I had a new pair of glasses, I could do some more reading.' My mother had macular degeneration and had been declared legally blind. When she eventually agreed to go into a nursing home at age 95, she said to me sternly: 'Why are you putting me in here with all these old people?' She never considered herself to be old.

Rather than letting Mum become sedentary in the nursing home, which was their culture, I would visit her three times a week and take her for a 1km walk. These walks retained her leg strength, which helped her avoid falls. Her positive attitude was also essential. I would like to think that I have inherited some of her positive genes, and that I will also stay healthy and positive into my 90s.

Retirement is not in my vocabulary

In 1988, I had left my position as Director of Planning and Community Development at Leichhardt Council with a staff of 120, and Vicki and I had established Gary Shiels and Associates. The company was a planning and traffic consultancy, which we started from home and as our staff grew, we moved the practice to an office in Paddington. Like any business we had numerous teething problems, although we grew to having 15 staff in Paddington and an office of five on the Gold Coast. Our company was very successful, and we were being engaged to assist with an increasing number of aged care facilities. As business partner and co-director, Vicki was critical to ensuring that the company maintained good cash flow and was financially viable. Although you work long hours when you own the business, you have some flexibility to fit in a gym or swim session. While I enjoy training with a group, I am quite relaxed in my own company. Perhaps this came initially from being an only child, and latterly because there are not many people around my vintage, who enjoy pushing themselves. Accordingly, I have no difficulty exercising vigorously by myself.

During COVID and reflecting on the past 33 years as Managing Director, I decided it was time for a further change. In 2021, aged 75, I stepped down as MD, although I retained the original company name of Gary Shiels and Associates, and worked as a consultant to the company. I then served as an Acting Commissioner in the Land and Environment Court and then, chair and expert member, on five Local Planning Panels determining development applications. Prior to and since moving on from GSA, Vicki has developed remarkable skills as an artist, with her work being widely admired by friends and colleagues, particularly her studies of horses and landscapes.

The word retirement is not part of my vocabulary. I prefer to think of this stage of life as a time to pursue meaningful projects and stay fully engaged. I have established a not-for-profit website, Successful Ageing with Dr. G (https://www.successfulageing. com.au/), which took a considerable amount of time and energy. The purpose of the website is to promote successful ageing, the benefits of exercise and a healthy Mediterranean diet, while avoiding refined/processed food. I have also made a number of presentations on healthy ageing, some with close friend and colleague, Dr John Best. This book has also taken considerable time and energy.

My evolving *ikigai*

In 2023 I was recognised in the Australia Day Honours List, when I received an AM for services to town planning, my commitment to lifesaving and working with the community. This award came out of left field, and I was both honoured and humbled. As I turn 80, I continue to practise what I preach. I exercise once or twice a day for one to two hours and do my best to maintain a healthy diet. Being as fit and healthy as I can be allows me to keep doing the things I love – like skiing in Japan and competing in surf ski races and the 1km soft sand race at the Masters championships. These activities are all part of what the Japanese call *ikigai*: my 'reason for being' or 'purpose in life'.

Monday morning starts at 5.50am, with Dr G's Ab Lab, when I take a squad of about 12 keen people and put them through stretching, Pilates, and some serious abdominals; this is followed by coffee. I have been running these classes at the surf club for almost 30 years. Other mornings start with either a 2km swim (three days a week with a squad), followed by Pilates; or on alternate days a 4km run on the soft sand (three days) followed by a sauna and a quick surf. I also ensure I fit in at least two weight workouts, as I believe maintaining strength and muscle mass is critical as you age. A couple of hits of golf and a massage tops off the week. There might also be a ski paddle on nice days or a game of pickleball. I don't know how I ever had time to work six days a week and go to uni. I hasten to add; people don't need to be as committed or obsessive as I am!

I believe if more people truly understood the quality-of-life benefits that come from regular exercise, they'd be more inclined to commit. Likewise, if they knew the health risks associated with many refined foods, they might think twice about what they put in their mouths.

In the next chapter we shall look at the marvellous instrument known as your body: its evolutionary origins, how our changing demographics affect society's health profile as a whole, various risk factors to our health, how we can maintain muscle mass and strength, how biological age is more important than chronological age, as well as the various ageing curves … and the importance of getting on the right one.

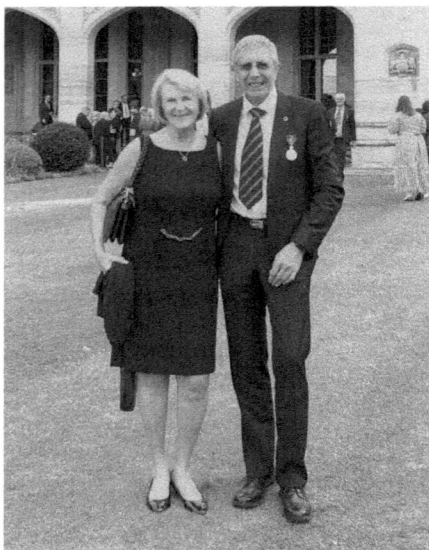

With Vicki, receiving the Order of Australia Medal at NSW Government House, in 2023.

CHAPTER 2: LOOK AFTER YOUR BODY

The amazing human body

The human body is truly remarkable. From when we are born until we die, the human body goes through a greater metamorphosis than any other animal on this planet. Our bodies are designed to move and be active and this can be traced back 60-70,000 years with the evolution of species from Neanderthals, who were mainly carnivores, to Homo sapiens, who were hunters and gatherers. In fact, the diet of both Neanderthals and Homo sapiens varied greatly, depending on where they were living and the food sources available. Neanderthals were also thought to have resorted to cannibalism when food was scarce, and the lack of zinc found in their teeth at one campsite would suggest they were high-level carnivores.

The Darwinian theory describes the evolution of the species and the survival of the fittest. The Homo sapiens, who outlasted the Neanderthals, were healthier, fitter and more adaptable which gave them a greater chance of survival.[23] The fitter they were, the better able they were to feed their families and defend themselves. Although we now see ourselves as civilised – even cultured – the same law of survival applies. The healthier and

---

23 Harari, Y.N. (2011). *Sapiens: A brief history of humankind*. Vintage Books.

fitter we are, the greater our chances of avoiding disease, enjoying a high quality of life and extending our health span.

The complexity of this structure in which we live never ceases to amaze me. Leonardo da Vinci (1452-1519 AD), who is said to be one of the greatest biological investigators of all time, was renowned for his drawing of the human figure. His drawing represents the proportions of the human body as a physical and spiritual entity.

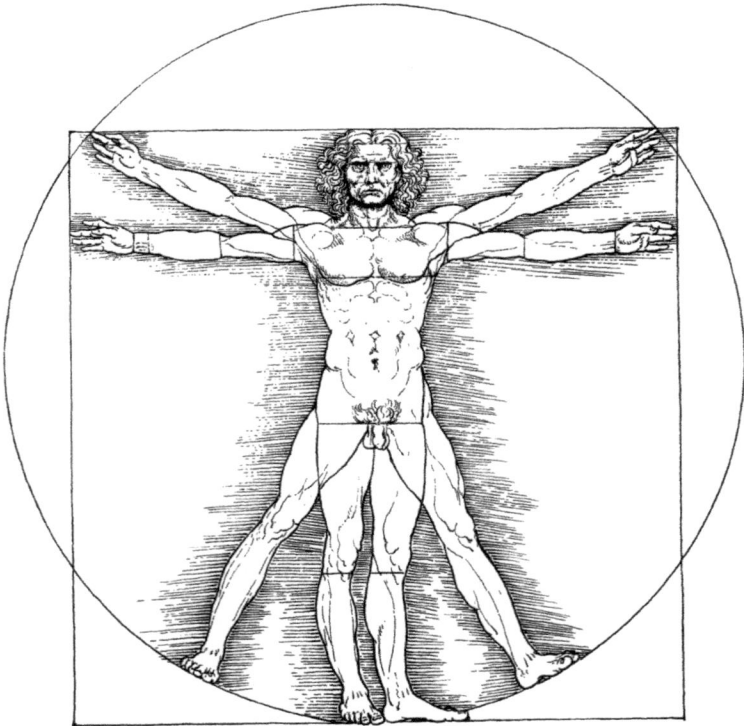

Figure 2.1: Leonardo da Vinci – Vitruvian Man, circa 1490. Source: Wikimedia Commons.

On a daily basis, the human body takes 23,000 breaths and has 100,000 heart beats, both of which are essential to our survival. These breaths and heart beats enable us to move the 600 skeletal muscles, that have a range of functions from pumping blood and supporting movement to lifting heavy weights or giving birth.

The human body is incredibly intricate, containing trillions of cells that take many forms and perform different functions. There are 36 trillion cells in the male body and 28 trillion cells in the female body. The human brain contains approximately 171 billion cells, with roughly 86 billion neurons and 85 billion other cells, primarily glial cells. These cells, including neurons and non-neuronal cells, work together to form the complex network that allows the brain to function.

The many types of cells in the human organism include stem cells, red blood cells, white blood cells, neutrophils, eosinophils, basophils, lymphocytes, platelets, nerve cells, neuroglial cells and muscle cells.

Based on where they are found, the function of the human cells can be divided into stem cells, bone cells, blood cells, muscle cells, fat cells, skin cells, nerve cells, epithelial cells, sex cells and cancer cells. While human cells contain a number of major parts, which play an important role in the body's function, we will concentrate on two parts that relate to ageing successfully: the nucleus and the mitochondria.

The nucleus acts as the cell's control centre, primarily responsible for storing and protecting the cell's DNA, which contains the genetic information. It also co-ordinates cellular activities like growth, metabolism and reproduction. It houses the cell's hereditary material (DNA) and directs protein synthesis.

The mitochondria, often called the 'powerhouses of the cell', are responsible for generating the majority of the cell's energy through a process called cellular respiration. They convert nutrients like sugars and oxygen into adenosine triphosphate (ATP), the main energy-carrying molecule used by the cell. Beyond energy production, mitochondria also play roles in cell signalling, cell growth, and even programmed cell death.

Insulin is stored in the pancreas, specifically within the beta cells of the islets of Langerhans. These cells produce and release insulin into the bloodstream in response to rising blood glucose levels. While the pancreas is the primary site of insulin storage and release, the liver and muscle cells also play a role by storing excess glucose as glycogen, a process facilitated by insulin.

Our cells are continually replaced, and this allows us to recover from an extensive range of activities/exercise and diseases. Cells can also be converted to the 'dark side' and become cancerous. We should be trying to feed our mitochondria and keep our metabolism and cells as healthy as possible as we age.[24] The potential downside of not looking after our mitochondria and metabolism is discussed in Chapter 8.

The heart and lungs are the engine rooms in our body and the way we treat them influences our health, including organs, brain, joints and bodily functions. If we fill our lungs with

---

24 Pleil, J.D., Ariel Geer Wallace, M., Davis, M.D., & Matty, C.M. (2021). The physics of human breathing: Flow, timing, volume, and pressure parameters for normal, on-demand, and ventilator respiration. *Journal of Breath Research*, 15(4), 10.1088/1752-7163/ac2589. https://doi. org/10.1088/1752-7163/ac2589

smoke, it will adversely impact on our organs, which makes us more vulnerable to a number of cancers and heart disease. We perform more efficiently if we have fresh air to breathe, water to hydrate, healthy food for nutrition, regular exercise, and sleep to recharge and cleanse our brains. Unfortunately, most of us fail to complete one or more of these sustaining tasks on a regular basis.

Australia has one of the longest life expectancies on the planet. Yet for many, health span does not equal lifespan and the last 10 to 20 years of life is spent without health and vitality. While we have never lived longer, observations would suggest that we have never felt sicker. According to the late American physician Dr Walter Bortz, who taught medicine at Stanford University and promoted the possibility of a 150-year lifespan, 'we spend too much time dying and not enough time living'.[25] More than half of our population, either unknowingly or unwittingly, are pursuing a lifestyle that promotes unwellness, disability, cancer or some form of disease. As we are living longer, it is critical that we respond to our changing demographic profile so that more people can enjoy a high quality of life in their later years.

Our changing demographic profile

The demographic profile of the Australian population has been consistently changing over the past 100 years, and these changes are predicted to continue. This profile has changed as a result of two World Wars, the Great Depression, the post-war baby boom and more recently the COVID-19 pandemic.

---

25 Bortz, W. (1991). *We live too short and die too long*. Bantam Books. (Bortz, 1991).

Two actual and a projected demographic profile for 1925, 2000 and 2045 show how dramatic this transformation has been, and it is projected to change even further in the next 25 years. According to Australia's Productivity Commission (PC), the age distribution is being squeezed into different shapes by our reduced fertility rates, ageing population and other demographic pressures.[26] The age structure of the Australian population moved from a 'pyramid' in 1925 to a 'beehive shape' in 2000 and is projected to resemble a 'coffin' by 2045. Hopefully, the unfortunate term used for the projected 2045 profile is not a metaphor for our ageing patterns in Australia. An extract of the diagrams reflecting these changing profiles is shown in Figure 2.2.

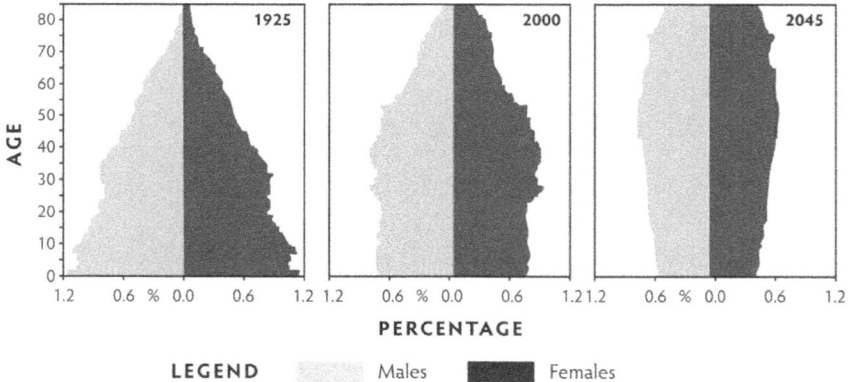

Figure 2.2: From Pyramid to Coffin: Changing Age Structure of the Australian Population, 1925-2045. Source: *Economic implications of an ageing Australia*. Productivity Commission Research Report, March 2005.

---

26 Productivity Commission. (2005). *Economic implications of an ageing Australia*. Productivity Commission Research Report. Australian Government. https://www.pc.gov.au/inquiries/completed/ageing/report/ageing.pdf

What this figure shows is that Australia's demographic profile is projected to become even more top heavy with increased numbers of older people and decreased numbers of younger people. The number of Australians aged 85 years and over is projected to double by 2042, increasing to over 1 million people according to the ABS.[27] The projected profile strengthens the need for our ageing population to be healthier and age well.

Our health issues

In Australia, 66% of the population is either overweight or obese. (In the US, by comparison, the number sits at about 73% of the population).[28] Yes, you read that correctly – two in three Australians are either overweight or obese. Since 1995, the number of people in Australia living with obesity has increased from one in five (19%) to one in three in 2022 (32%).[29] As mentioned previously, one in three Australians aged over 70 take five or more different medications.[30] We are told by the medical profession that increased medication is to be expected as we age. It has been suggested, by some, that ageing is a disease and that disability and decrepitude is the natural progression we should expect. I don't subscribe to that theory. As the New Age writer Marilyn Ferguson observes, 'of all the self-fulfilling

---

27 ABS. (2018). *Population aged over 85 to double in the next 25 years.* https://www.abs.gov.au/articles/population-aged-over-85-double-next-25-years

28 AIHW. (2024). *Overweight and obesity.*; National Centre for Health Statistics 'Obesity and overweight' https://www.cdc.gov/nchs/fastats/obesity-overweight.htm

29 AIHW. (2024). *Overweight and obesity.*

30 Quek et al., 2025.

prophecies in our culture, the assumption that ageing means decline and poor health is probably the deadliest'.[31] There are many diseases that can kill us, but ageing, of itself, is not one of them. I support the Jack LaLanne model and the Dr Walter Bortz doctrine of 'use it or lose it!' My belief is most of us can control the manner in which we age. We just need to recognise and avoid the lifestyle risk factors and be cautious of the culture of any aged care facility we are considering for relatives or ourselves.

Many aged care facilities thrive on the myth that we should do less as we age. It is more cost effective if residents are inactive and sit or sleep for long periods during the day. It requires more staff, and costs more money, to keep older people fit and active. But the fact of the matter is that there is a greater need for exercise as we get older. So, if you are considering an aged care facility for yourself or a loved one, look for a high level of programmed physical activity as a criterion.

Nutrition is equally important. As we age, we have an increased need for nutrition as our bodies are less able to absorb vitamins and minerals from the food we eat. Our diets have changed dramatically, and not for the better. We consume insufficient vegetables and fruit, and an increasing number of sugary drinks and refined food (see Chapter 6). If an aged care facility has poor quality food and encourages a sedentary lifestyle, it is a lethal combination. Being inactive and consuming inadequate amounts of fruit and vegetables accelerates biological ageing past our chronological age and provides a less fulfilling

---

31 Ferguson, M. (2009). *The aquarian conspiracy: Personal and social transformation in the 1980s.* Tarcher.

lifestyle in the twilight of our life.

The characteristic being more widely recognised as a primary behavioural risk factor of ageing is being sedentary. The risk of Alzheimer's disease is also much greater for sedentary people. Without exercise the blood travelling to the brain is not flushed regularly, providing greater opportunity for a build-up of plaque and disconnections in the brain.

Being sedentary is now acknowledged by the World Health Organization (WHO) as one of the causes for a number of diseases. WHO research has found that regular physical activity reduces risk of many types of cancer by 8-28%; heart disease and stroke by 19%; diabetes by 17%, depression and dementia by 28-32%. It is estimated that 4 to 5 million deaths per year could be averted if the global population was more active.[32] Instead, many older people feel they should do less as they age. While you may not want to hear this, the opposite is true. You need to *do more, not less* as you age. Most long-lived people are active, vital and enjoy healthy longevity into their 80s, 90s and beyond. Countries like Japan have more centenarians than other countries. Why are we not enjoying these health outcomes in Australia?

Risk factors

As part of my research, I interviewed 20 health professionals (half medical and half non-medical) who worked with older people. The medical experts included some of the most eminent in

---

32 WHO. *Physical activity.* https://www.who.int/health-topics/physical-activity#tab=tab_1

Sydney, that specialise in different parts of the human anatomy. The specialisations included a brain surgeon, psychologist, psychiatrist, cardiologist, prostate surgeon, gastroenterologist, gerontologist and my GP. The non-medical included a sports physiologist, a nurse, a massage therapist and an aged care provider. I asked them to identify the behavioural and biomedical risk factors that they most frequently observed in their patients, in order of priority. Their responses are summarised collectively below.

Behavioural

Their collective opinions were that being sedentary was the most frequently occurring behavioural risk factor and, in their opinion, it was the most dangerous. The second-most frequently identified risk factor was an unhealthy diet, which translates to insufficient consumption of fruit and vegetables, and a high consumption of processed food and sugary drinks. ABS data confirms approximately 95% of Australian adults do not consume the recommended levels of vegetables and fruit. Among 55-64 year olds, 4% met it; among 65-74 year olds, 6% met it; and among the 75+ group, 8% met it – an indication perhaps of 'survival of the fittest'.[33] (The recommended intake, of course, is two serves of fruit and five serves of vegetables.[34]) The third risk factor was insufficient sleep, thereby not allowing the body to

---

33 ABS. (2023). *Dietary behaviour*. https://www.abs.gov.au/statistics/health/food-and-nutrition/dietary-behaviour/latest-release

34 Heart Foundation. *Fruit, vegetables and heart health*. https://www.heartfoundation.org.au/healthy-living/healthy-eating/fruit-vegetables-and-heart-health

detoxify and replenish itself. The next two – drinking excessively and smoking – are ongoing problems in society. Others include socio-economic factors, and vitamin and mineral deficiencies. The behavioural risk factors identified in my interviews with health professionals are included in Figure 2.3.

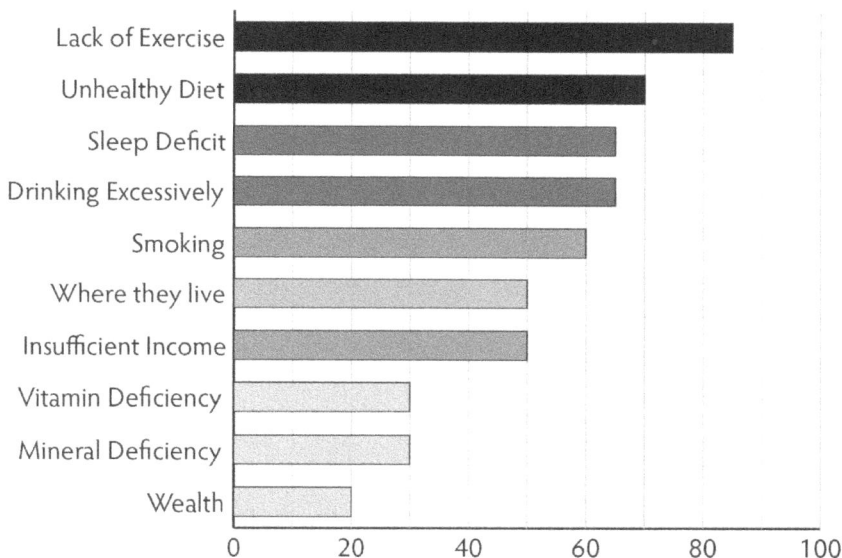

Figure 2.3: Ten most frequent behavioural risk factors of patients. Source: Author's interview responses from health professionals.

Biomedical

When our bodies are subject to behavioural risk factors, e.g. being sedentary, or a collection of risk factors, our mind and body respond, and we suffer from downstream effects which are known as biomedical risk factors. The biomedical risk factor most frequently identified by health professionals was overweight and obesity, which is often related to being sedentary and other behavioural factors that might include diet.

Surprisingly, depression was a close second in the biomedical risk factors identified. Whether it was a cause or effect was a matter for debate among the health professionals I spoke to. A psychiatrist I interviewed observed that a few of his patients with depression were suffering from a cluster of biomedical risk factors and being treated with polypharmacy. The research shows that depression is linked to overweight and obesity, diabetes, high cholesterol, high blood pressure, and high blood sugar – in fact, all of the identified biomedical risk factors. Most frightening is that these biomedical risk factors are often the precursor to heart disease and multiple forms of cancer. For most of us, if we control our behavioural risk factors, we can control our biomedical risk factors. The biomedical risk factors identified in my interviews are included in Figure 2.4.

My argument is ageing is not the disease argued by some authors, and you can avoid the behavioural and biomedical risk factors. The disease is not moving or being sedentary. Maintaining muscle mass, strength and VO2 is critical for ageing well. (VO2 max is the maximum rate of oxygen consumption attainable during physical exertion and will be discussed below.)

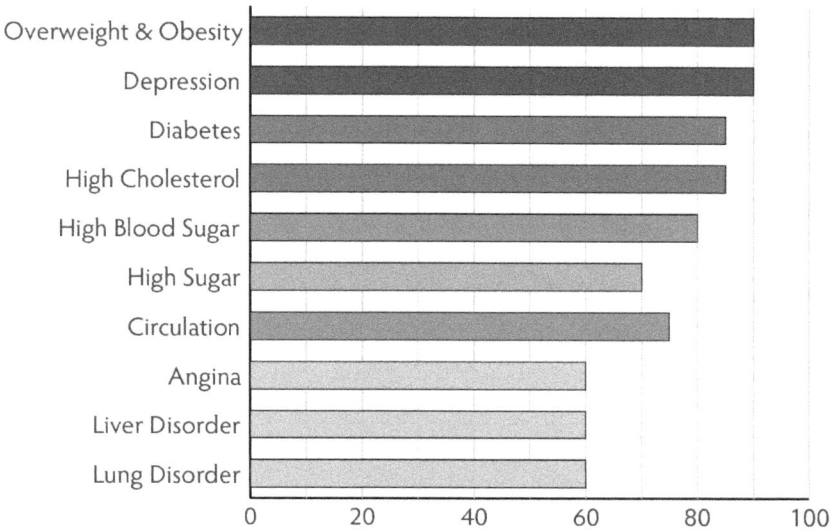

Figure 2.4: Ten most frequent biomedical risk factors of patients. Source: Author's interview responses from health professionals.

Maintaining muscle mass, strength and VO2

Many older people believe that ageing means decline, disability, disease, decrepitude and dependency (what I call the 5 'Ds'). If they are sedentary, they are probably correct. A sedentary older person is likely to have a reduced grip strength, be short of breath and have difficulty walking up a hill or stairs.

There are many tests of our biomarkers to measure health and longevity. Two simple tests are strength and VO2 max. A sedentary person can lose 3-5% of muscle mass per decade after the age of 30 and as much as 40% by the time they are 80. If an older person is sedentary, their muscles atrophy, resulting in a loss of muscle mass and a loss of muscle strength. The loss of strength is even greater than the loss of muscle mass. With the loss of muscle mass and strength, sarcopenia and a loss of bone density is inevitable, followed by osteoporosis and frailty, together with the likelihood of falling. If someone with this condition falls and breaks a bone or a hip, there is a poor chance of them recovering. Incredibly, one in four people who break their hip will die within 12 months.[35] Even if they recover from the fall, the bed rest and further muscle atrophy that follows is likely to be fatal. Also, a sedentary person normally has a less active immune system and therefore has greater vulnerability to disease and cancer.

A loss of strength equation for a sedentary older person might be expressed as follows:

Loss of strength ▸ decreased activity ▸ vulnerability to disease ▸ frailty ▸ dependence ▸ isolation

If we challenge this equation of inevitable decline in strength, adjust the equation, and change the values, we can get a totally different result. By replacing sedentary ageing and inactivity with successful ageing and increased activity, there can be improved strength, improved physical health and vigour, independence and greater stability, and a lowering of the biological age.

An increase in strength equation for an active older person might be expressed as follows:

---

35 Australian Commission on Safety and Quality in Healthcare. (2023, 11 September). *Time to surgery is critical for survival after hip fracture* [Media release]. https://www.safetyandquality.gov.au/newsroom/latest-news/time-surgery-critical-survival-after-hip-fracture#_edn2.

Increased strength ▸ increased activity ▸ improved health ▸ vigour ▸ independence ▸ lowering of your biological age

At any age you can improve strength, which will improve physical performance generally, and in the process help to slow down your biological clock and the ageing process. As early as 1638, Galileo noted that there was a direct relationship between body mass, physical activity and bone size. At my age, I was able to rebuild muscle mass and strength after recovering from two lots of shoulder surgery. It was not an easy process, and it does take real commitment. However, it is doable. I will discuss this in more detail when I deal with rehabbing the body in Chapter 8. However, it is important to remember that you won't get a different result by doing the same thing! If you have not been getting the muscle mass retention or development you are seeking, you probably need to change your exercise program.

The heart is the main part of the body we need to look after. It goes without saying smoking or vaping is high risk behaviour, and potentially lethal to boot. The heart is a vital muscle, and like any muscle in the body, it needs to be exercised. Again, our sedentary person, who is not exercising, has more exposure to cardiovascular disease (CVD) and cancer, likely weight increase and premature death. The test frequently used by cardiologists is a stress or VO2 max test.

The sedentary person's equation might be expressed as follows:

Reduced VO2 activity ▸ vulnerability to CVD + cancer ▸ potential increased body fat (30%) ▸ premature death

An alternative equation where increased activity becomes the driver for a healthy heart can provide a completely different set of results. The equation with changed values might be expressed as follows:

Increased VO2 activity ▸ reduced chance of CVD + cancer ▸ improved health span ▸ lowering your biological age

The WHO research confirms the extent of heart disease and cancer that could be prevented if we could encourage people to exercise. It is never too late to start, and exercising will help keep you above the disability threshold, which I will now discuss.

Disability threshold

The disability threshold is a level of health and fitness, identified by WHO, to describe a theoretical line that a person falls below when they are no longer able to care for themselves.[36] The WHO diagram, which I have modified to include my three ageing curves, indicates when each of the three ageing curves fall below the disability threshold. The typical ageing curve crosses the threshold late in mid-life and assistance in some form will be required. The optimistic ageing curve crosses the threshold late in older life. The successful ageing curve stays above the disability threshold almost until the end of life. I hasten to add this is a hypothetical interpretation that can vary from one person to another. A diagram showing the relationship of these curves to the disability threshold is shown in Figure 2.5.

36 WHO. (2002). *Active ageing: A policy framework*. https://extranet.who. int/agefriendlyworld/wp-content/uploads/2014/06/WHO-Active-Ageing-Framework.pdf

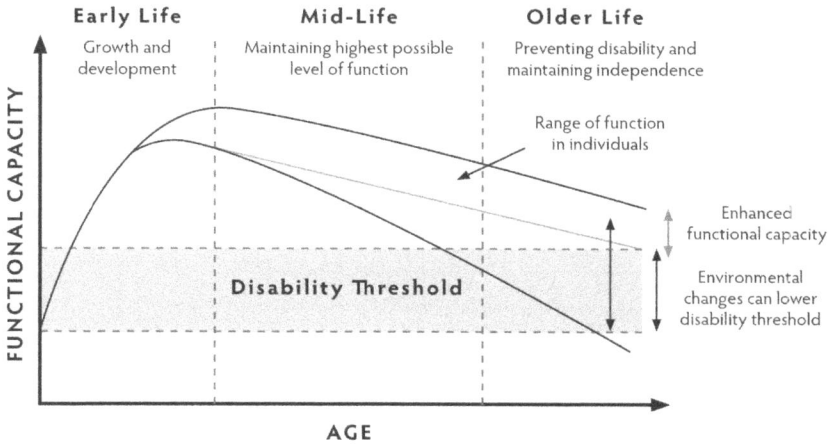

Figure 2.5: Adjusting the Disability Threshold and maintaining functional capacity over the lifetime. Source: Adapted from WHO, *Active ageing: A policy framework*, 2002.

Choosing your ageing curve

Research by Paffenbarger and Olsen suggests there are three potential survival curves that may describe the way we age.[37] These survival curves are also referred to in the literature as ageing curves, or life curves. My three ageing curves and my estimate of the percentage of the population under each curve are as follows:

- The typical ageing curve, which is typical of an estimated 60-70% of the population and the manner in which they age.
- The optimistic ageing curve, which includes an estimated 20-30% of the population, who avoid the majority of risk factors.

---

37 Paffenbarger & Olsen, 1996.

- The successful ageing curve includes an estimated 10-20% of the population and are those who avoid all of the risk factors.

My curves modify the earlier work by Paffenbarger and Olsen in four respects – adjusted curve descriptions, updated lifespans, and the inclusion of medication and disability zones. The medication zone occurs when people are likely to require prescribed medication, and the disability zone is when people can no longer care for themselves. My positive approach is to encourage everyone, who can, to pursue the optimistic or successful ageing curves and remain above the disability threshold as long as possible. Let's discuss these ageing curves in more detail.

The typical ageing curve

The typical ageing curve fits the profile of 60-70% of the population and relates to someone who has taken a number of behavioural risks and as a result now has biomedical problems. The typical or usual pattern for ageing is often a result of a number of both behavioural and biomedical risk factors that I mentioned in the previous chapter and frequently include things such as having a sedentary lifestyle, being overweight, having a poor diet, being sleep deficient and/or being substance addicted. If you are sedentary, a smoker or have three or more risk factors, then you may fit within the usual ageing curve. As mentioned, the usual curve is typical of our population, and has been described as resembling a ski slope, with declining health and vitality that begins early and results in premature death, typically from cardiovascular disease or cancer. The two shaded areas in the next graph, that I have referred to as the medication and disability zones, normally become part of life at an earlier age and can impact on health span and quality of life. The medication treatment continues through the disability zone. While these zones are arbitrary, they are indicative of someone on this profile. Today, medication has assisted in extending the lifecycle considerably, and many people may have prolonged life in the medication and disability zones. As we observed, two in three (66%) Australians are either overweight or living with obesity. This percentage increases among older Australians – a peak of 81% among males aged 65-74 and a peak of 70% for women aged 55+. The number decreases in the 75+ cohort – with 74.2% of males and 69.1% of females overweight or obese.[38] This decrease is mainly due to the fact obese people normally do not live as long as people who are not overweight. Studies show that obese people can expect to live 10 years less than people of a healthy weight. This typical ageing curve, with theoretical medication and disability zones, is shown in Figure 2.6.

---

38   AIHW. (2024). *Overweight and obesity.*

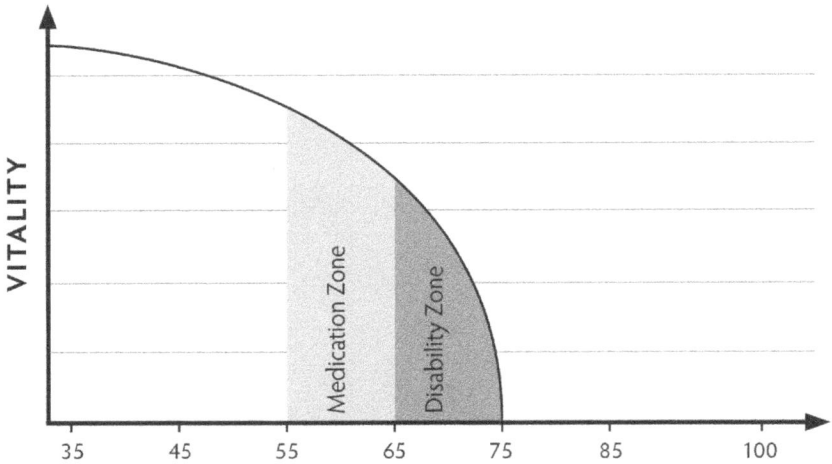

Figure 2.6: The Usual/Typical Ageing Curve. Source: Author's compilation.

The optimistic ageing curve

The second curve is described as the optimistic ageing curve, where the level of decline is less than the typical ageing curve. This ageing curve defers the need for medication and assistance until later in life. People on this curve, as shown by the red line in Figure 2.5, are likely to remain above the disability zone for a much longer period of time. A lifestyle akin to this second ageing curve has the potential to provide a greater quality of life than the typical curve. A lifestyle with less behavioural risk factors is likely to result in less biomedical health problems and the deferment of disease and disability until much later in life. If you have avoided the behavioural risk factors, are a healthy weight and have, say, two or less of the biomedical risk factors (and you are not overweight or living with diabetes), then you might be within this ageing curve as shown in Figure 2.7.

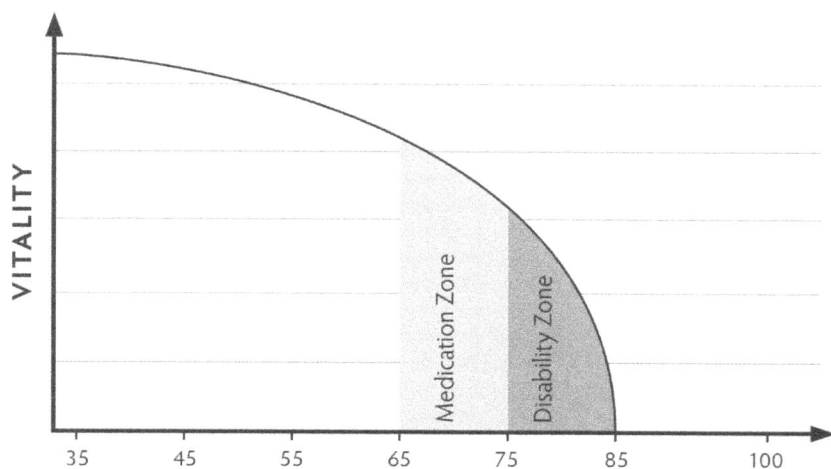

Figure 2.7: The Optimistic Ageing Curve. Source: Author's compilation.

The successful ageing curve

The final diagram shows the successful ageing curve, where a person avoids all of the risk factors and retains a high level of strength and fitness throughout life. Instead of a gradual decline, the ageing curve is almost rectangularised, which enhances the quality of life, extends the lifecycle and, importantly, extends the health span, where health span (almost) = lifespan. This successful ageing curve theory also postulates that the time spent in the medication and disability zones can be deferred or minimised to the near end of life and morbidity can be compressed. This successful ageing curve is shown diagrammatically in Figure 2.8.

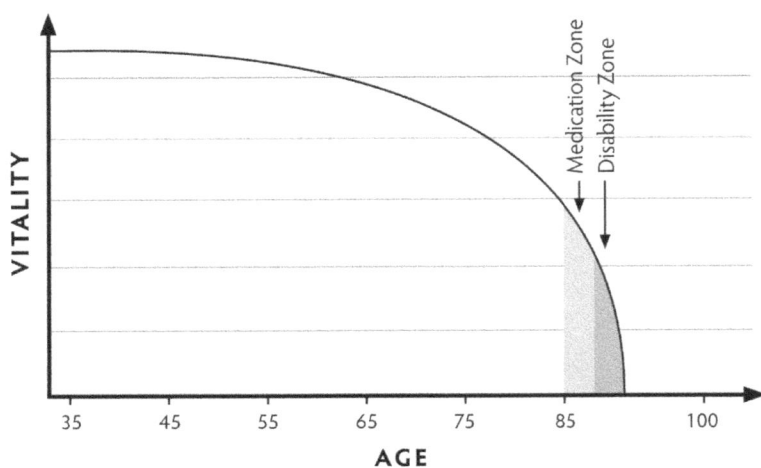

Figure 2.8: The Successful Ageing Curve. Source: Author's compilation.

Dr John Rowe, a geriatrician physiologist, and Dr Robert Kahn, a social psychologist and co-author with Rowe of the book *Successful Ageing* (1998), were part of a 10-year study for the MacArthur Foundation to examine why people age differently. They were endeavouring to distinguish between the concept of successful ageing from, what they described, the usual pattern of ageing, considered to be part of the ageing process.[39] In their theory, an older person with optimum health could avoid disability and disease. The concept of successful ageing places emphasis on limiting behavioural and biomedical risk factors, while promoting a healthy and nutritious diet and physical activity, thus creating the potential for retaining physical and mental function. The Rowe & Kahn Model of successful ageing contains three characteristics:

---

39 Rowe, J.W. & Kahn, R.L. (1998). *Successful Aging*. Pantheon Books. (Rowe & Kahn, 1998).

- low risk of disease and disease-related disability;
- high mental and physical function; and
- active engagement with life.

These can be shown diagrammatically in the following Figure 2.9.

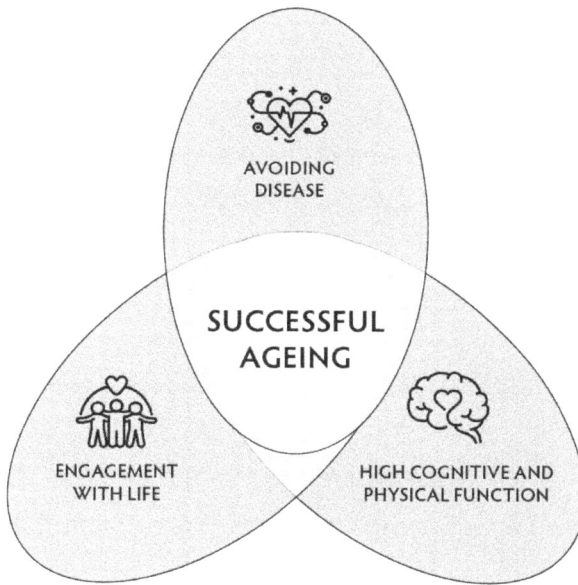

Figure 2.9: Components of Successful Ageing. Source: Adapted from Rowe & Kahn, 1998.

Rather than spending months or years struggling with disease or disability or living in a nursing home or in palliative care, the aim of successful ageing is to rectangularise your ageing curve and compress morbidity, with deferred or eliminated disability, until near death. As discussed in the introduction, the critical elements of my Successful Ageing Paradigm are as follows:

1. Your chronological age is irrelevant; it is your biological age which is important; and you can lower your biological age.
2. Attitude, activity, adventure, appreciation and associations (the five As) are your new lifestyle; 60 is the new 40; 80 is the new 60; and 100 is the new 80.
3. Decline, disability, decrepitude, disease and dependency (the five Ds) are not mandatory or inevitable; and ageing is not a disease.
4. Enjoy the pleasures of the moment without dwelling on the past or being overly concerned about the future. Many miss the pleasures of the now, worrying about the past or future.
5. Establish your short-, medium- and long-term goals, then prepare your own personal exercise program (PEP) that will achieve those goals.

In the next chapter, we shall look at the famed Blue Zones – places where people live to 100 and more – the diet and lifestyle that allows them to become centenarians and supercentenarians, how this lifestyle slows ageing, as well as meet the Elders: 20 long-lived people, who I interviewed who are models of ageing successfully.

Before you read on, pause and ask yourself two questions:

1. **Which one of the three ageing curves best describes your current health and lifestyle?**
2. **Which one of the three ageing curves would you be prepared to commit to moving forward on?**

CHAPTER 3: THE BLUE ZONES

There have been many stories and considerable research to identify the longest-lived people on the planet. An early fictional story by English writer James Hilton spoke of Shangri-La, which was described as the land of the immortals. Sadly, Shangri-La centenarians are fictional, however other media reports in the 1970s highlighted areas where people lived extraordinarily long lives. Some of the areas identified included Abkhazia, the Hunza Valley, Vilcabamba, and Okinawa. In these areas it was suggested that there were centenarians and supercentenarians (aged over 110), and it was early research by US physician and research scientist Dr Alexander Leaf that tested some of these claims.

Dr Alexander Leaf

Dr Alexander Leaf was a professor in clinical medicine at Harvard University and Chief of Medical Services at Massachusetts General Hospital. Although he did not believe in the fountain of youth, he made a study of long-lived people. Research by Dr Leaf published in the *National Geographic* magazine drew international attention to very old people in three remote communities undertaking high levels of physical activity and fitness.[40] These older people were actively farming and tilling the ground, performing strenuous tasks, at what we would describe

---

40 Leaf, A. (1973). Every day is a gift when you are over 100. *National Geographic*, vol 143, issue 1. 93–118.

as old age. People of this age in Australia are normally sedentary and/or in nursing homes.

Dr Leaf's studies included observations of people in the Abkhazia region in the Caucasus mountains of the then USSR; the Province of Hunza Region in the Karakoram Mountains of north-western Pakistan; and the isolated village of Vilcabamba in the Andes Mountains of Ecuador. Dr Leaf focused on the Abkhazians in the Caucasus mountains as he thought they must be the longest-lived people on the planet with claims of lifespans well over 100 and achieving 110, 130, and even 150 years of age.

Dr Leaf noted that sickness was not considered a normal or natural event even in the very old. He recorded interviewing an Abkhazian Elder who was nearly 100, who had good hearing and 20/20 vision. Dr Leaf asked the man if he had ever been sick. The man replied that he once had a fever. When Dr Leaf asked the man if he had ever seen a doctor, the man replied, 'No, should I?' Dr Leaf noted the man had blood pressure of 118/60 and a pulse rate of 70 bpm. A blood pressure measurement in this range, by our standards, is considered to be excellent at any age, and uncommon without medication.

He concluded that the lifestyle in these communities was the common factor in their vitality at 80-100 years of age and more. Obesity in these regions was extremely uncommon. Although there was moderate consumption of alcohol and tobacco, many biomedical risk factors were absent and there was very little incidental disease and cancer. Dr Leaf also observed that diets were low in calories and animal fats, with high consumption of plant-based food, coupled with high levels of physical activity. The terrain in these regions contributed to the need for strenuous exercise.

People in these regions were mainly vegetarians and vegetables were normally raw or cooked in a very small amount of water. Vegetables were normally picked just prior to a meal, to ensure that the food was totally fresh. Nuts including almonds, pecans, beechnuts and hazelnuts form an important part of almost every Abkhazian meal.[41] In contrast in modern society, preservatives, sprays and refrigeration are used to extend the shelf life of fruits and vegetables. Not to mention our heavy reliance on animal protein, processed food and fast food.

Another factor highlighted in the research was the incredible respect for the aged, which was a distinctive feature of the culture. In Abkhazia, a person's status increases with age, and he or she receives greater privileges with the passing of years. Elders are respected and revered, simply for getting older. Instead of being called 'old people' they are referred to as 'long-lived people.' Which brings to mind something US President John F. Kennedy said in 1960: 'The treatment of its older citizens is said … to be one of the most basic tests of how civilized a society or nation has become.'[42]

While Dr Leaf considered that Abkhazia deserved its reputation as the mecca of super longevity, subsequent research found that claims for extraordinary long lives were not well

41 Robbins, J. (2006). *Healthy at 100: How to extend your life and stay fit!* Hodder & Stoughton. (Robbins, 2006).

42 John F. Kennedy Presidential Library and Museum. https://www.jfklibrary.org/archives/other-resources/john-f-kennedy-speeches/washington-dc-19600126

documented and could not be substantiated. Although the long-lived Abkhazian Elders were vital and heathy with health spans close to their lifespans, their ages may have been enhanced to receive the additional recognition that comes with every passing summer.

With a few exceptions, the Vilcabambans and Hunzans have similar lifestyles to the Abkhazians and pursue a vegetarian diet. The Hunzans have exceptional apricot orchards and attribute their longevity to their consumption of apricots.

People in each of Dr Leaf's long-lived cultures enjoyed some form of alcoholic beverage. However, they did not indulge to excess and only drank in moderation.

Dan Buettner

Another *National Geographic* correspondent, explorer Dan Buettner, travelled to many locations around the world with a team of scientists to examine the components for longevity.[43] An internationally recognised researcher, explorer and *New York Times* bestselling author, Buettner identified five geographic regions where individuals lived exceptionally long and healthy lives, longer than the average life expectancy. From the acknowledgments in his book, Buettner seems to have been influenced by the 2001 research by Willcox et al., identifying Okinawa as having the longest-lived people, rather than the earlier observations by Dr Leaf. I will discuss the Willcox et al. research later in this chapter. The Buettner-identified regions also had the highest concentrations of centenarians.

---

43 Buettner, D. (2008). *The Blue Zones*. National Geographic.

Buettner described these locations as 'Blue Zones' in reference to the concentric blue circles previous scientists had drawn on a map to highlight areas where people lived longer lives. These zones are shown in Figure 3.1 and include the following locations – Nicoya, Costa Rica; Ikaria, Greece; Okinawa, Japan; Sardinia, Italy; and Loma Linda, California.

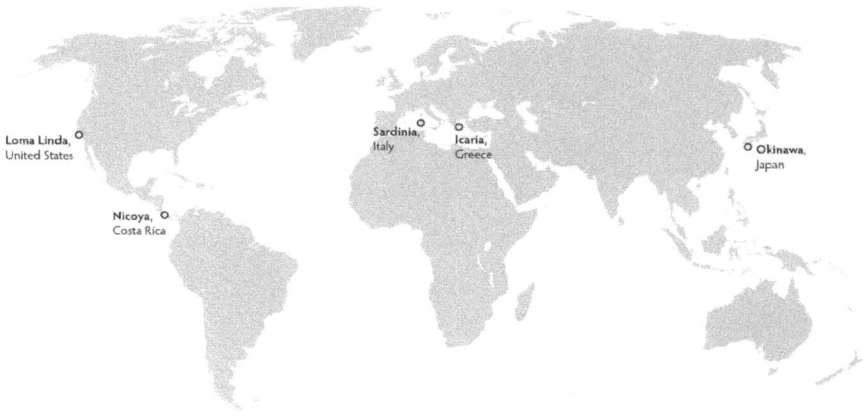

Figure 3.1: The Blue Zones (Adapted from www.bluezones.com)

Blue Zone diet and lifestyle

The diets and lifestyles of the Blue Zone populations vary from one region to another. However, there are many commonalities. In Nicoya, Costa Rica, for example, squash, corn and beans form the foundation of the traditional diet. On the other hand, people in Ikaria, Greece, tend to follow a Mediterranean diet emphasising whole grains, beans, potatoes and olive oil. However, these populations also share some of the following common characteristics.

Eat in moderation

People in Blue Zones tend to consume small- to moderate-portioned meals, which helps them to maintain a healthy body weight. You may have heard this described as the '80% rule', eat until your belly is 80% full. In Japan, this rule is known as *hara hachi bu*. This rule or phrase, described as the Okinawan Mantra, is inspired by Confucius, and is often said before or after meals to remind one to only eat moderately and avoid overindulgence. How would this be received in the Australian household? It may not be popular, but it would be a healthy innovation.

To achieve *hara hachi bu*, the Japanese serve themselves moderate portions. That means no seconds and no super-sizing. To reduce portion size, they use smaller plates rather than a full-size dinner plate. They also eat no more than three meals a day and don't snack between meals. This helps to explain why Japan has the least number of obese people. A member of my Monday morning Ab Lab sessions recently lost 30kg, without medication, by simply improving the quality and reducing the quantity of the food he consumed, together with a bit more exercise. He mainly avoided sugar, bread and processed food, and ate more vegetables. According to him, it really was quite simple!

Follow a plant-based diet

A Blue Zone diet typically consists of whole, unprocessed foods high in nutrients and low in unhealthy fats and sugars. Plant foods such as fruits, vegetables, legumes, beans, nuts and wholegrains are all staples. These foods are packed with vitamins, minerals and antioxidants that can help protect against disease and promote overall health. Furthermore, Blue Zone diets may include lean proteins such as fish, poultry and eggs, but red meat is rarely consumed. Dairy products also are limited or avoided altogether.

Live actively and with purpose

People in Blue Zones get a lot of physical activity but it's generally not from going to the gym. They are active in their daily lives. For example, someone in a Blue Zone might walk or cycle to get from one place to another rather than commute by car. Also, the traditional Japanese lifestyle includes very little furniture: they sit, eat and sleep on the floor and their everyday life involves continually getting up and sitting down on the floor. If you try this for a day, you will appreciate the strength and dexterity required. They do this every day, which enhances their balance and flexibility.

Often, Blue Zone jobs and hobbies are active as well. For example, sheepherders in Sardinia, Italy, walk at least five miles a day as they traverse mountainous terrain. In Okinawa, Japan, most people tend gardens daily, growing produce they consume and share with their neighbours. In Nicoya, Costa Rica, people find purpose and joy in completing daily physical chores such as sweeping, walking to various destinations, tending to cattle and hand-washing their clothes.

Know your reason for being

In Okinawa, there's a saying, *ikigai*, which translates to 'purpose of life'. If you have not read the book *Ikigai*, you should, it is a great read. Similarly, in Nicoya, Costa Rica, the phrase *plan de vida* translates to 'soul's purpose' or 'life plan'. People who live in these communities are not merely trudging through the day. Instead, a deep sense of purpose gives them a reason to wake. When coupled with a strong sense of community and faith, this sense of purpose likely helps buffer stress. It also may help to keep people active as they age.

To strengthen your *plan de vida* consider activities that would allow you to contribute to your community. Like the Okinawans, could you tend to a garden and share produce or flowers with your neighbours? Or perhaps you could learn a new skill or help someone with their chosen career skills. If you're a teacher for example, you might volunteer to tutor local children. Or, if you work in healthcare, you might offer your skills at a non-profit clinic. Finally, if you're active in a faith community, you might volunteer in that capacity. There are many ways to pursue your *ikigai*.

How does the Blue Zone lifestyle slow ageing?

Blue Zone diet and lifestyle modifications work together to help you maintain a healthy body weight, which, in turn, can help you live longer. It really is not rocket science – just avoid refined food, consume plenty of vegetables, reduce the portion sizes, and move more in your day-to-day activities.

A nearly instant fix to overweight and obesity is to move to a plant-based diet with moderate portions. It will reduce the number of calories you consume. Purposeful physical activity (which is where I started and will talk more about in subsequent chapters), helps you increase the number of calories you burn. It is easier said than done, of course. Which is why researchers also suggest developing a renewed sense of purpose that can help to draw you closer to your community, buffer stress and find a reason to live a healthier life.

The Okinawa Program

Bradley Willcox, Craig Willcox and Makoto Suzuki are longevity researchers best known for their book *The Okinawa Program* (2002), which explores the lifestyle and dietary habits of Okinawan Elders known for exceptional health and lifespan. Their work blends epidemiology, gerontology and cross-cultural health insights to promote successful ageing worldwide. Their book, which was based on a 25-year study, confirmed that Okinawa has the longest-lived people, and Japan has the greatest number of centenarians.

After examining over 600 Okinawan centenarians and numerous 'youngsters' in their 70s, 80s and 90s, they observed clear patterns were emerging. In particular, it became obvious that the Okinawan lifestyle was providing some real, scientifically verifiable reasons why these people were incredibly healthy in their very senior years. Dr William Osler, known as the father of modern medicine, once observed that 'a man is only as old as his arteries'.[44] The same can be said of a woman. Our arteries are our lifelines; if our blood circulation is compromised in any part of the body, we are at risk of injury or death. The Okinawan

---

44 Willcox, B., Willcox, C., & Suzuki, M. (2002). *The Okinawa Program*. Harmony.

centenarians had arteries like 20- and 30-year-olds. High blood pressure (hypertension), a common problem in Australia, was almost non-existent among the Elders in Okinawa. Similarly, there were few incidents of heart attacks or strokes and other diseases or cancers. It really makes you think! What are we doing wrong?

The study concluded that it was the lifestyle determinates that were responsible for their successful ageing, specifically regular exercise, diet, moderate alcohol use, avoidance of smoking, stress minimisation and spiritual outlook. Bradley Willcox and colleagues found that Okinawans were at low risk for hormone-dependent cancers, in particular breast, prostate, ovarian and colon cancers, compared to Western society. The lifestyle determinants they identified included mainly diet – low caloric intake with high consumption of soy, vegetables and fish; moderate alcohol; high levels of physical activity; and low body fat.

Their diet included fish three times a week (usually oily fish), a variety of plants and nuts, and a considerable amount of fibre with a limited amount of red meat.

Okinawans also had strong social networks, referred to as the Moai. These community groups were family and extended family, who looked after each other. If one member of this extended family fell on hard times, the group would band together to provide food, shelter or whatever was needed.

The China Study, the promise of the future

One of the most comprehensive studies on nutrition ever conducted, The China Study, began in 1983 and is still going. In the 2005 book by T. Colin Campbell and Thomas M. Campbell,[45] they arrived at some interesting revelations about diet. However, their respective backgrounds are worth briefly summarising.

T. Colin Campbell, PhD, is a nutritional biochemist renowned for his research on the link between diet and disease, and a professor emeritus at Cornell University. Now in his 90s, he is the lead author of The China Study. Thomas M. Campbell, MD, is a physician and researcher specialising in nutrition-based preventative medicine. He co-authored The China Study with his father, T. Colin Campbell, and is a leader in plant-based health advocacy.

In particular, they concluded they could see the benefits produced by eating a plant-based diet are far more diverse and impressive than any drug or surgery used in medical practice. They further observed that heart diseases, cancers, diabetes, strokes and hypertension, arthritis, cataracts, Alzheimer's disease, impotence and all sorts of other chronic diseases can be largely prevented.

These diseases, which generally occur with ageing and tissue degeneration, kill the majority of us before our time. They concluded that a plant-based diet could avoid many of these diseases, that are otherwise linked to normal ageing. Importantly,

---

45 Campbell, T. C. & Campbell, T. M. (2005). *The China Study*. BenBella Books.

they argued that many of the drugs currently recommended by the medical profession could be avoided.

China's records of long-lived residents are not well documented, which was part of the reason for The China Study. The landmark research compared the full Chinese range of diets – diets rich in plant-based foods to diets very rich in plant-based foods. In almost all other Western studies, scientists were comparing diets rich in animal-based foods to diets very rich in animal-based foods.

Rural-based Chinese diets and Western diets had different disease patterns. The China Cancer Atlas, which was part of the research, provided mortality rates for more than four dozen different kinds of disease and presented a rare opportunity to study the many ways that people die. Interestingly, The China Study also identified diseases of poverty and diseases of affluence. At the time of the study, Western diseases of affluence were not common in regions where a plant-based diet was consumed. The diseases of poverty were a result of nutritional inadequacy and poor sanitation, while the diseases of affluence were a result of nutritional extravagance.

We can learn from the lifestyles of these long-lived communities to help us to avoid the unhealthy influences in Western society.

The Elders

A critical part of my research involved interviewing 20 long-lived people between the ages of 80 and 104 who were, prima facie, healthy and ageing successfully. The average age of the Elders was 86 and collectively they had lived 1,710 years. I selected

80 as the youngest age limit as that was beyond the average lifespan of males in Australia when I commenced my research. As I am now in my 80th year, I realise it is just another number and my argument continues … chronological age is irrelevant, what's important is your biological age and that's what we need to work on.

I selected my candidates using a snowball sampling technique with sources providing the name of older people who might meet my criteria. I refer to my candidates as Elders, as a mark of respect, and I was looking for participants who were ageing exceptionally well, or as I prefer to say, ageing successfully.

The Elders came from different backgrounds. Those still working included: a developer, an architect, a ski instructor and a physical training instructor who trained older people. A number of the Elders were performing voluntary work, assisting other older people or helping a spouse with daily duties. The majority of interviewees lived in the Sydney metropolitan area with a few from western Sydney, one from the Central Coast and one living in Queensland. For privacy reasons, any reference to the Elders was, and will be, by first name only. Research has found that a positive attitude to ageing results in greater durability and an additional 7.5-year lifespan.[46] With one exception the Elders had avoided the behavioural and biomedical risk factors expected in old age. The exception had heart disease, which he said was a wake-up call that changed his life.

---

46 Levy, B.R., Slade, M.D., Kunkel, S.R., & Kasl, S.V. (2002). Longevity increased by positive self-perceptions of aging. *Journal of Personality and Social Psychology*, 83(2), 261–270. https://doi.org/10.1037//0022-3514.83.2.261

In a self-assessment of physical and mental health, widely recognised as an acceptable method of measuring health, almost all of the Elders considered themselves to be of excellent or good health, with only one suggesting they were of average health, namely the Elder with heart disease. None of the Elders identified themselves as being in poor or fair health, which is in contrast to a national self-assessment survey, where only one third of over 75s rated themselves as being of excellent or very good health.

Generally, around half of Australians aged over 15 (56.4%) consider themselves to be in excellent or very good health, while 14.7% reported being in fair or poor health.[47] The frequency of exercise that the Elders were pursuing was astonishing. Three in four (75%) did some form of physical activity seven days a week. This level of commitment is exceptional by any standard. A few pursued physical activity five times a week, while one Elder pursued exercise four days a week. All Elders pursued physical activity at least three days a week.

The overwhelming attitude of Elders was positive, with a positive self-image and an optimistic outlook their common attitude to life. They were not controlled by technology and seemed to take life as it came, and they were stress-free. The concept of *Yutori* helps to explain the Japanese psychological state of sufficiency and ease – and it helps me explain how the Elders I interviewed appeared to me to be. They seemed not to be overwhelmed or underwhelmed, and they were making time for things that they considered to be meaningful.

---

47 ABS. (2018). *Self-assessed health status*. https://www.abs.gov.au/statistics/health/health-conditions-and-risks/self-assessed-health-status/latest-release

All of the Elders were of the opinion that they consumed a healthy and balanced diet, advising that they had fruit and vegetables on a daily basis. The Elders also had a variety of intellectual pursuits and had extensive support networks. Sleep was an important factor, with all of the Elders averaging between seven and nine hours a night. A synthesis of their recommendations for successful ageing included: a positive attitude, pursuing physical activity, healthy sleep patterns, eating healthy food, remaining socially connected, having a purpose in life and avoiding risk factors. In effect, the Elders had developed their own blueprint for successful ageing, and their collective lifestyle components for successful ageing are shown diagrammatically in Figure 3.2.

Each interview was different, and I was incredibly privileged that these outstanding Australians made time for me and provided me with their personal insights as to why they had aged so remarkably well. Although I have maintained confidentiality for each of the Elders, I've included some deidentified information about them below. This will give you a flavour of what they did to create their own blueprint for successful ageing, which helped to ensure they had a successful and enjoyable life in their later years.

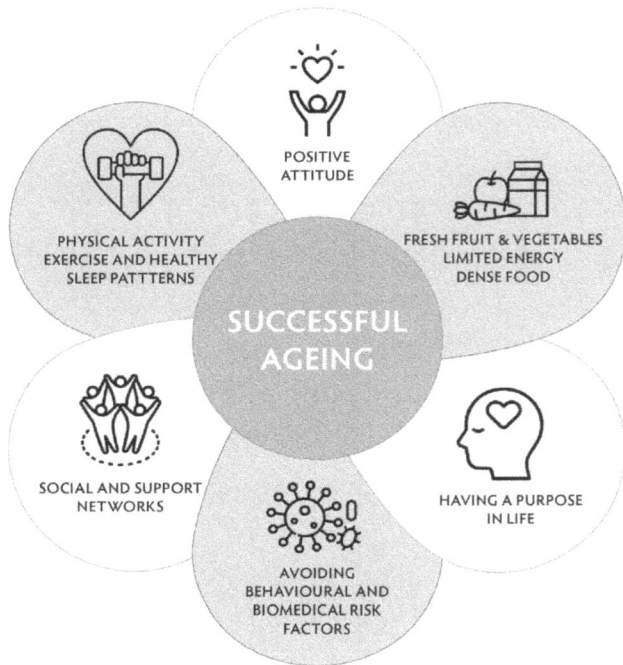

Figure 3.2: Elders components for Successful Ageing. Source: Author's compilation.

Victor – *The lean, mean running machine*

Victor was a lean and fit 80-year-old when I interviewed him as part of my research. He was 180cm tall, weighed 70kg and was either running, swimming or bike riding seven days a week. Victor was living with, and caring for, his wife in a seniors housing development. His wife had suffered a stroke and had advanced dementia. In spite of Victor's circumstances, he described his life as having 'a lot of satisfaction' and his attitude as 'an attitude of gratitude'. Victor's amazing philosophy on life was, 'If it is to be, it is up to me'. Victor had already lived beyond the average life expectancy at that time for males in Australia and was atypical of his age cohort, who were overweight, sedentary and taking numerous forms of prescribed medication.

Victor appeared to have a fitness level and mental acuity of a fit 50-year-old. Why was Victor ageing successfully and his much younger wife incapacitated? Was it Victor's positive attitude, diet or devotion to exercise that was the secret to him being physically fit, mentally acute and amazingly positive? I believe so. Victor was living proof that vigorous exercise helps us to live a healthy life and avoid cancer and disease that is synonymous with ageing. If we are prepared to commit to a healthy lifestyle, successful ageing can be the enduring benefit.

Victor's Blueprint for Successful Ageing is characterised by his amazingly positive attitude. His vigorous exercise every morning set him up for the day, which would sometimes be challenging, with the decline in health of his wife. Their accommodation ensured nutritious food, and a good circle of friends.

Nancy – Lived to serve others

Nancy was an amazing 104-year-old who was still mobile, articulate and living in a nursing home. Nancy had enjoyed an active life and even at her age was still walking and exercising every day. She was located in one of the better nursing homes that encourages older people to be active and engaged. Nancy volunteered to assist nurses and staff on a daily basis in the nursing home, and the staff allowed her to pursue these voluntary activities. The staff appreciated that this was Nancy's purpose in life.

Nancy's Blueprint for Successful Ageing was created by her kind heart, and the tolerance of the aged care staff who allowed her to feel she was an integral part of the team carrying out important duties.

John – Astute businessman

John was 81 years old when I interviewed him. He was, and still is, a very successful businessman. He was exercising daily, swimming 500m and walking 6km. He lived in an impressive house in Sydney's Eastern Suburbs with his wife of many years. He enjoyed his exercise, had a healthy diet, an insatiable intellectual appetite and was an avid reader. He also had a strong social network of friends and associates. I see John on occasions: he has turned 93, still exercises daily and is still living in the same house, which is close to services and facilities. His wife has now moved to a nursing home.

John's Blueprint for Successful Ageing is notable for his determined attitude, daily exercise, healthy lifestyle, strong purpose and close network of friends.

Grant – A life spent on the slopes and the beach

Grant was 81 when I interviewed him, in good physical and mental condition and, as a single man, virtually lived two lives. In the Australian winter, he worked as a ski instructor in Perisher, in the Australian snowfields. In the Australian summer, up until he turned 80, he took ski tours to Austria, where he would guide skiers around the Austrian Alps. In summer, when he was home, he lived in a small semi in Bondi and would be at the surf club most days, doing some exercise and chatting with his mates. He was affable, had a particularly positive attitude, and nothing seemed to worry him. He would always greet you with his welcoming smile and friendly comments, which made you feel good that you had seen him. He never had a negative word to say about anyone. He had the happy knack of always being able to enjoy the moment.

Grant made a great speech at his 90th birthday at Perisher, which I attended. After thanking the many friends who had attended his party, from all over the planet, he said, 'You only come this way once, but if you do it well, once is enough!'

Grant's Blueprint for Successful Ageing was to enjoy the moment and always remain positive. Grant passed away at 92.

Dr Bill – *Outstanding athlete, party animal and businessman*

A close friend of mine, Dr Bill, is a retired general surgeon. I interviewed him in his previous role as a health professional. Bill has also been a top-level athlete, having played 100 first grade rugby league games. He has run a few marathons, competed in numerous triathlons and is still a very competitive skier. The pinnacle of his sporting achievements was winning his then-age group (50+) in the Hawaiian Ironman. For those who may not be familiar with this event, which is total insanity, it consists of three legs: an open water 3.86km swim in Kailua-Kona Bay; a bike ride over the Hawaiian lava landscape 180.25km to Hāwī and back; and a 42.19km marathon run along the coast from Keauhou to Keahole Point and back to Kailua-Kona. After the event he spent a few days on a drip recovering.

Dr Bill has also been through some hard times and after retiring as a general surgeon, remarrying and making a good investment, he is back to a very strong financial position.

To celebrate his 82ⁿᵈ birthday, Bill and I skied non-stop for three-and-a-half hours in Thredbo in the Australian snowfields. We then stopped at Kareela Hutte, halfway up Crackenback Mountain, for lunch, which involved copious quantities of wine and excellent food (not recommended on a daily basis!). Bill continually reminds us that he 'loves having a good time!' There would be few 82-year-olds who party like a 20-year-old and ski like a fit 40-year-old.

Dr Bill's Blueprint for Successful Ageing includes having a home he loves, a healthy diet and a strong network of friends. Bill is still active, and his positive attitude has been the catalyst for his success.

Harry – The affable golfer

Harry was an inspiringly fit 92-year-old. He arrived at the surf club gym at 5am on a daily basis, walked the 4km to Bronte and back, did a weight session and finished his workout with a dive in the surf at North Bondi. Harry referred to his dive into the ocean as his visit to see Dr Bondi.

Harry was also still playing very competitive golf at least three times a week and was upset that his handicap had drifted out to about 20 in later years. (This is a handicap that 70% of golfers would be happy to have!) I recall him arriving at the gym one morning with his legs bandaged quite heavily.

Thinking it may have been an older person's fall, I enquired about his injury. He advised that he had been playing golf at his beloved Bonnie Doon golf course in nearby Pagewood when his playing partner had hit his ball into the rough. Unless you have observed the rough at the Doon you may not appreciate the experience. Harry explained how he climbed into the rough, looking for his friend's ball, only to be caught up in the spinifex. He fell onto the path, causing the injury. There would be few 92-year-olds who would be able to play golf, let alone go hunting for a lost ball in spinifex.

Harry was an affable person, with an outstanding memory. He would walk into the surf club gym each morning and greet everyone by their first name, seldom getting it wrong. He would also have a few words of encouragement for everyone he greeted. He was a classic example of geriatrician Dr Walter Bortz's theory – *use it or lose it.*

Essential to **Harry's Blueprint for Successful Ageing** were the surf club visits in the morning, the nursing home where he lived with his wife, and his golf club.

• • •

In summary, you can create your own blueprint for successful ageing wherever you live. If you maintain your health, wellbeing, strength and mental acuity, until near death, you can create your own blueprint for successful ageing wherever you live.

In the following chapter we will observe that a positive attitude is the habit we need to develop. It doesn't happen naturally for most people; however, it is a habit you can cultivate. We will consider our centenarians in a bit more detail, and I will introduce you to a number of role models who inspire positivity and have provided me with inspiration.

Before you read on, pause and ask yourself two questions:

1. **If you knew you could create your own blueprint for successful ageing right where you live, would you make the effort?**
2. **Are you prepared to change your lifestyle?**

CHAPTER 4: A POSITIVE ATTITUDE

People born with a positive attitude are most fortunate. They have the confidence that invariably leads to success in the things they pursue. A positive attitude is also a catalyst for getting out of bed in the morning. It helps you commit to exercise, a nutritious diet, and it provides you with the confidence to maintain your social networks. People with a positive attitude are also better able to solve problems as they are continually looking at other options to find a solution. As we observed, studies have shown that having a positive attitude results in a longer lifespan. Accordingly, we should all aspire to have a positive attitude.

However, not all of us are brimming over with confidence and we need to work at being positive. A quote attributed to Aristotle supports this idea: 'We are what we repeatedly do, therefore, excellence (or positivity) is not an act, but a habit.'

Similarly, James Clear, motivational speaker and productivity expert, describes in his 2018 book, *Atomic Habits*, a four-step process he calls 'the habit loop', which I believe we can use to train ourselves to think more positively. These four steps are: Cue – observing something we find inspirational/attractive (retailers continually provide us with cues to sell us items); Craving – a feeling that we would like to be somewhere, or do something (we are frequently influenced by a cue to buy or do things); Response – the feeling of achievement from pursuing a task (the cue has provided the craving, which resulted in the response); and Reward – the feeling of satisfaction having completed the task or helped someone (having responded to the cue and the craving, our reward is to be satisfied with our actions).

When something becomes a habit, it becomes our natural reaction or our default position. According to Clear, we can apply this habit loop to everything we do: our studies, at work, pursuing physical exercise or developing our social skills. Taking a positive approach can also become a habitual way to deal with life's challenges.

Conversely, a terrible experience in life can influence our attitude. Perhaps it may break us, but then again, maybe it will make us more determined – the choice is up to us. Viktor Frankl, during his time as a prisoner in Auschwitz, showed that everything can be taken from a man except one thing – the last of the human freedoms is the freedom to choose one's attitude in any given set of circumstances, to choose one's own way. Frankl regularly observed to his patients and students in Vienna, it was something he had to go through alone, without any help and it inspired him for the rest of his life. Like Frankl, our attitude to life and living can be instilled by a traumatic experience. Regardless of our approach, we need to practice positivity until it becomes a habit.

This chapter considers the benefits of having a positive attitude to life, particularly as it relates to ageing. It includes the stories of four incredible centenarians and other role models who I have been fortunate to know, or know of, who changed my life, and will hopefully have a positive impact on you.

Australian centenarians and supercentenarians

Catherina van der Linden – *Supercentenarian*

Catherina was born in the Netherlands on August 26, 1912, and was believed to be the oldest living Dutch person in the world. Catherina migrated to Australia with her husband and young family in 1955. The mother of four worked as a grape picker, nursing assistant, typist and clerical assistant, and inherited a love of fashion from her mother.

Catherina moved into Southern Cross Care's West Beach Residential Care home in South Australia in 2019, and soon became a healthy ageing role model for fellow residents.

In August 2023, before she passed away, Catherina was quoted as saying: 'I push myself sometimes when I'm getting a bit tired and I think it's about time to do something to yourself to see that you still have that energy that you had before. I still go on the bike, sometimes for 10 minutes and that is a long time to spend on the bike.'

A spokeswoman in the nursing home where she lived said Catherina became a healthy ageing role model for fellow residents, with her love of regular gym sessions and walking. She credited her longevity to her active lifestyle.

When asked on her 111th birthday in August 2023 what was her advice for a long life, she replied, 'be happy and be content with what life gives you … and of course keep moving, don't sit still'. She attributed her longevity to being active.

Catherina van der Linden passed away on Australia Day 2024 in South Australia at age 111, and at that time, was Australia's oldest person.

Catherina founded her **Blueprint for Successful Ageing** in an environment where she lived and thrived, firstly in her neighbourhood and then in the nursing home. She prioritised exercise, eating healthy food and staying connected to many friends.

Ken Weeks – Supercentenarian

Ken Weeks has been officially confirmed as the oldest Australian man, at 112 years, recently taking Catherina's title as the longest-lived person. Ken lives in an aged care facility in Grafton, NSW. Born in 1913, he was the eldest of five children born to Darcy and Dorothy Weeks. As a child, he attended Grafton High School.

In 1941, at the start of World War II, Ken married Jean McPhee (1911-1986); the couple had two sons, Ian and Noel. They were married for 45 years before Jean's death in 1986.

Ken had many occupations throughout his working life, working on construction jobs like building roads and constructing wartime airfields at Evans Head. He was also a truck driver, a petrol station operator, and an employee at the Grafton match factory. He was also a co-owner of a Chrysler car dealership and repair business in Grafton. During World War II, he applied to join the Royal Australian Air Force (RAAF), but at a height of just 1.5m, his short stature led to him being turned away. After World War II, he set up a radio and electrical sales and repair business in Grafton, which he operated for several years before later replacing it with a milk bar. He eventually worked as a school bus driver in Clarence Valley, before ultimately retiring at the age of 65.

He attributes demanding work, a happy life and having a purpose for his longevity. He also credits his long life to a healthy diet, which includes baked beans. Ken started eating baked beans more than 30 years ago and when he turned 110, Heinz did a special edition can of baked beans to celebrate his birthday. Ken also says he has no regrets in life.

Ken created his **Blueprint for Successful Ageing** in Grafton where he lived, then in the nursing home where he still lives. He remains active, and on last reports, he was still walking without a walking stick. His diet still includes baked beans, and he remains connected to friends.

Dr Gladys McGarey – *Centenarian*

Dr Gladys McGarey was born in 1920 in India and was a truly remarkable 103-year-old, referred to as the mother of holistic medicine. As you might expect, she had many recommendations for healthy longevity. Gladys always had an active outdoor life and had to walk a mile to and from school every day, which included a 300m incline in the Himalayas. She moved to North America with her parents, where she studied medicine and set up a practice for holistic medicine.

Gladys recalled in a recent interview: 'I started exercising as a child, and never stopped, and I still have a daily step count.'[48] Gladys was an omnivore and ate all sorts of foods:

---

48 Mooney, J. (2024). How to live to 100: Longevity lessons from 103-year-old Dr Gladys McGarey. *Body+Soul*. https://www. bodyandsoul.com.au/health/health-news/how-to-live-to-100-longevity-lessons-from-103yearold-dr-gladys-mcgarey/news-story/ f3a968ab4eab94558701cc2a26d4cad1

meats, vegetables, carbs and proteins. However, she avoided processed foods and tried to have a salad with some chicken at lunch and a smaller meal at evening. Gladys observed that having a purpose in life, learning something every day, and trying to find the humour in difficult situations eases tension. A massage every week and enjoying each day was important for her to have a fulfilling life. Gladys was actively pursuing her passion of holistic medicine from 1940 until she passed in September 2024.

Gladys created her own **Blueprint for Successful Ageing** with a focus on helping people and keeping active.

Peter Manner – *The running chef and centenarian*

Five years ago, I was part of a wine tasting tour to the Hunter Valley in NSW, and I was impressed by one of the senior members of our touring team. Peter Manner was 95, thoroughly enjoying a glass of wine, and he was particularly mobile. We started chatting and he told me that he was living by himself and still enjoyed cooking. He was as sharp as a tack. Peter advised that he had only stopped running the City2Surf two years earlier. He began running the event when he was 73 and completed 20 events before deciding he had had enough.

Peter was an unassuming, polite, entertaining gentleman, who swam at least 500m every day. He was a recognised chef amongst his peers. I had the pleasure of attending his 100th birthday. He died in 2025, aged 101. Peter's positive attributes for a healthy older age included enjoying the moment and pursuing challenges at any age.

Peter created his own **Blueprint for Successful Ageing** where he lived, where he exercised, and where he met up with friends. He always enjoyed the moment.

Well-known role models with a positive attitude to ageing

Next are five well-known role models – two living, three deceased – who showed an exceptional approach to ageing well.

Sir Richard Branson (1950 –)

For many years, I have admired the courageous business acumen of Sir Richard Branson and the staff at Virgin, who are always incredibly positive. Initially, Branson set up his own company, Virgin Records, and then later established Virgin Airlines. Recently, reading a story about how Sir Richard lives his life, and leaving aside his professional success, I appreciated that we had a few things in common. Sir Richard, now 75, was not overly committed at school. He has been married for approximately 50 years and was close to his mother, who passed at 96.

For the last 30 years he has been a keen exerciser and trainer, spending up to three to four hours a day on fitness. He is conscious about his diet, eats healthy food, limits his alcohol intake, goes to bed at 9pm, gets up at 5am and tries to get a good night's sleep. Also, he likes to push himself and meet challenges, just to show he can do things that many people much younger cannot. Importantly, his major emphasis is to enjoy each day rather than worrying about longevity. Of course, the major difference between us is our bank accounts and investment portfolios.

Sir Richard creates his own **Blueprint for Successful Ageing** wherever he goes and whatever he pursues.

Jane Fonda (1937 –)

Jane Fonda, born on December 21, 1937, in New York City, is an acclaimed American actress, political activist and fitness advocate. The daughter of legendary actor Henry Fonda, Jane Fonda began her acting career in the 1960s, achieving significant success in films like *Klute* (1971) and *Coming Home* (1978), for which she won Academy Awards.

In the early 1980s, Fonda embarked on a new venture: promoting fitness and healthy living. She released her first exercise video, *Jane Fonda's Workout*, in 1982, which became a cultural phenomenon and helped revolutionise home fitness. Her workouts emphasised aerobic exercise, strength training and body awareness, making fitness accessible to millions of women.

Fonda's commitment to exercise and wellness has continued throughout her life. She published several books on fitness, nutrition and self-care, such as *Jane Fonda's Workout Book* and *Being a Teen*. Her advocacy for a healthy lifestyle included promoting mental wellbeing, emphasising the importance of a balanced diet, and encouraging regular physical activity.

Beyond fitness, Fonda has remained active in social and political causes, using her platform to support issues such as women's rights, environmental activism and anti-war movements. Today, at 87, she continues to inspire others with her lifelong dedication to health, fitness and activism, proving that age is no barrier to living a vibrant and fulfilling life.

Jane Fonda has created her own **Blueprint for Successful Ageing**, via exercise, a healthy lifestyle, positivity and social activism. In a recent interview she was quoted as saying, 'at 87, I feel younger and healthier than in my 20s'.[49]

George Burns (1896 – 1996)

George Burns is a great example of a positive approach to ageing. He was still doing stand-up comedy in his late 90s. His wit and advice on ageing were always well-received. Burns argued that too many older people practised being old. He would say, 'they think themselves into dotage by adopting what they consider to be expected mannerisms and lifestyles of the elderly'.

Burns argued that lifestyle should be short on inactivity and semi-dependence, and long on vigorous exercise and self-reliance. A testimony to his spontaneity and quick wit were his onstage responses to doting fans. George was asked by one fan, 'Is it okay to have sex in the 90s?' He responded quickly, 'I prefer to stop in the 70s, after that it tends to get a bit hot!' His trademark cigar formed part of his onstage performance, and he admitted to enjoying a glass or two of Scotch.

While Burns would make light of the ageing process, he was committed to encouraging older people to think young and remain active. He led by example as a role model for ageing disgracefully and passed away at 100.

---

49 Rocca, J. (2025, April 20). Jane Fonda: 'I was very old at 20 and feel quite young at 87'. S*ydney Morning Herald* https://www.smh.com.au/topic/jane-fonda-3h7

George Burns created his own **Blueprint for Successful Ageing** by enjoying himself and having fun – at home, on the stage, and through the image he portrayed on screen.

Kirk Douglas (1916 – 2020)

As a young lad growing up, I greatly admired the American actor Kirk Douglas (born Issur Danielovitch, in Amsterdam, New York). A robust athletic man with a distinctive character, he was able to play an amazing variety of roles over four decades on the silver screen. I was first impressed by his role in *Spartacus* (1960) where his athleticism was on display. His body of work included *Young Man with a Horn* (1950), *Gunfight at the O.K. Corral* (1957), *Paths of Glory* (1957), *The Brotherhood* (1968), *There was a Crooked Man* (1970), *The Man from Snowy River* (1982), *Tough Guys* (1986) and numerous others over a very distinguished career.

During my research I discovered Douglas's commitment to exercise. As he maintained that commitment, he enjoyed robust good health until suffering a stroke in 2002, at age 86. He remained active after his stroke and wrote a number of books, many best-sellers. His books included *My Lucky Stroke* (2002) and *90 Years of Living, Loving and Learning* (2007). Douglas died in February 2020 at age 103. He remains an example of someone who never gave up on life and went on to become an accomplished writer who was trying to help others by sharing his life experiences.

Kirk Douglas created his own **Blueprint for Successful Ageing** in life as a movie star, and as an author. He was committed to exercise and making the most of every opportunity.

Jack LaLanne *(1914 – 2011)*

Francois Henri 'Jack' LaLanne was an American fitness, exercise and nutritional expert and motivational speaker who was sometimes called 'the godfather of fitness' and the 'first fitness superhero'. Although I never met him, LaLanne remains one of my inspirational role models. He motivated millions of people to live a healthy and active life. As a teenager, he was not naturally gifted and dropped out of school because of ill-health. In a 2003 interview, he relayed his life story and spoke about being shy, having pimples and boils, being thin, weak, and sickly, and needing to wear a back brace.[50]

LaLanne recalled that he used to suffer from headaches and wanted to escape his body because he was constantly in pain and his life appeared hopeless.[51] Nutritionist Paul Bragg was the catalyst for changing LaLanne's approach to life, from eating cakes, pies and ice cream to consuming a healthy diet and pursuing exercise.

LaLanne set out to find out what he could achieve from a dramatically improved diet and the pursuit of exercise. LaLanne found a set of weights and started using them and also became meticulous about what he ate. He developed exercise equipment that evolved into what has become standard in many gymnasiums, fitness centres and health clubs in the US and Australia today.

---

50 Hughes, J. & Hughes, D. (2003). Interview with Jack LaLanne. *Share Guide*. www.shareguide.com/LaLanne.html
51 Robbins, 2006.

LaLanne opened the first health club in 1936 in Oakland, California, which would become the catalyst for the numerous types of fashionable gymnasiums that we know today. Many people thought he was a charlatan and could not be trusted – particularly when he encouraged the elderly to lift weights, contrary to doctors' advice. At the time, doctors argued that the elderly would have heart attacks and break bones. In fact, it has now been shown that the opposite is true.

He argued that weight bearing exercises were critical for building strength and preventing elderly bones from breaking. LaLanne was also one of the first to advocate strength training for women. As a religious man, he would ask when he prayed each evening: 'God, please give me the willpower to refrain from eating unhealthy food when the urge comes over me and give me the strength to exercise when I don't feel like it.' He also presented his ideas to millions of people on television in those early days, which helped many of them change the way they viewed health and fitness.

Jack LaLanne started life as a shy, bullied and introverted young person and became a committed – and eccentric – promoter of health and fitness. He did extraordinary things on his 60th, 65th and 70th birthdays. For example, on his 60th he swam from Alcatraz Island Prison to San Francisco, towing a 1000-pound boat. LaLanne said that his purpose for doing these phenomenal feats was to demonstrate that an active and healthy lifestyle can work wonders.

LaLanne was living testimony to the value of regular exercise and a healthy lifestyle. He used to be vegan and late in life occasionally ate egg whites and wild fish, but mostly he ate organic raw fruit and vegetables and took a number of vitamin supplements. As noted previously, LaLanne's mantra was: 'Exercise is King. Nutrition is Queen. Put them together, and you have a Kingdom.' He and his wife, Elaine, spoke all over the world inspiring people to help them to a better life physically, mentally and morally. Jack and Elaine LaLanne were married for over 50 years.

Prior to his death, he was asked if he would like to live to 100. His reply was, 'I don't care how long I live! I just want to be living while I am alive!' LaLanne passed away at age 96 in 2011 from respiratory failure due to pneumonia.

Two testimonials recognised LaLanne's contribution to society. Actor and director Clint Eastwood, another long-lived person, said, 'Jack knew the values of exercise and nutrition before it became fashionable.' Bodybuilder, actor and politician Arnold Schwarzenegger said: 'Jack LaLanne was 30 years ahead of his time. He was truly the Terminator of unhealthy living. He possessed the secret formula for the fountain of youth.'[52] As a role model, LaLanne has had a profound impact on me, and he has inspired me to continually challenge myself. He was truly an inspirational person who has influenced my life.

Jack LaLanne created a **Blueprint for Successful Ageing** that has been adopted all over the world, and he led by example, showing that exercise and a healthy lifestyle can do anything.

---

52 On his Facebook page, Schwarzenegger also described LaLanne thus: 'Jack was literally an apostle for fitness, and his gospel inspired billions all over the world to live healthier lives.' https://www.facebook.com/arnold

Researchers in ageing

During the research for my PhD and these writings, I have read numerous books: however, several authors stood out as they were living their experiences, as indeed I am. The first three helped to enlighten my approach to ageing, while the fourth was written by a cancer survivor who became an athlete. Their contributions are summarised below.

Drs Rowe and Kahn – 10-year study of ageing

One of the earliest studies of ageing was sponsored by the MacArthur Foundation in the 1970s and 1980s over a 10 year period. It was conducted by Dr John W. Rowe, MD and Dr Robert L. Kahn, PhD. Dr Rowe was a geriatrician physiologist and the founding Director of the Division on Ageing at Harvard Medical School, while Dr Kahn was a psychologist and social scientist who was considered a pioneer in the fields of organisational theory and survey research. Together they also co-authored the book *Successful Ageing* (1998).

The goal of the study was to move beyond the limited view of chronological age and to clarify the genetic, biomedical, behavioural and social factors responsible for enhancing functionality in later life. Importantly, they concluded that ageing is not determined by genes alone and that lifestyle plays an important role. For example, they were examining what factors conspire to put one octogenarian on cross-country skis and another in a wheelchair. Considering that this study was undertaken over 50 years ago makes it even more groundbreaking at the time.

The positive results from this study influenced me considerably, and it is referred to throughout this book. The Rowe and Kahn positive approach to ageing has been one of the guiding lights for my research.[53]

Rowe and Kahn helped create the **Blueprint for Successful Ageing** for others, by showing in their research that the five Ds were not inevitable, and it was possible to age successfully in your own environment.

Dr Walter Bortz – *Use it or lose it!*

My early research was enlightened by Dr Walter Bortz MD, one of the most respected authorities on ageing. He was the former President of the American Geriatrics Society, and a Professor at Stamford University Medical School. Dr Bortz first described the term 'disuse syndrome' to describe how a lack of physical activity can destroy health, leading to premature ageing.[54]

Dr Bortz found that when people become sedentary, their entire physiology atrophies, resulting in the heart, arteries, and other parts of the cardiovascular system becoming vulnerable. Also, muscles and skeleton become frailer, obesity becomes a greater risk, and depression is often the end result. My interviews with health professionals found that depression was one of the most frequently occurring health risks for older people. What many people fail to acknowledge is that these premature symptoms for ageing are not a result of our chronological age;

---

53 Rowe & Kahn, 1998.
54 Bortz, W. M. (1984). The disuse syndrome. *Western Journal of Medicine,* *141*(5).

they are invariably a result of a sedentary lifestyle.

Dr Bortz identified the term which I live by today, 'use it or lose it'. His 1991 book, *We Live Too Short and Die Too Long*, identified the conundrum we are experiencing in present-day Australia. Although we are living longer than ever, for many people, the last 10 or 20 years of life is with chronic disease or disability. Not only does Dr Bortz describe how to achieve and enjoy a 100-year plus lifespan, but he also leads by example. In his mid-70s, Dr Bortz and his wife were still regularly running marathons. He says, 'for me, exercise is the sacrament of a commitment to living life fully'.[55]

Dr Bortz became committed to running at 40 years of age, to cope with the overwhelming grief of the death of his father. He ran the Boston Marathon at age 80 and continued running until age 86. As he approached his 89th birthday, he still maintained that setting goals and accepting challenges allowed him to be as alive and creative as possible. Indeed, goalsetting is his main recommendation for successful ageing. Dr Bortz is a role model who not only researches and writes but leads by example.

Dr Bortz created his own **Blueprint for Successful Ageing** by becoming committed to his own research and recognising the importance of exercise.

Dr Ralph Paffenbarger – *Choose how you age*

Dr Ralph Paffenbarger (Paff to his friends) was a sedentary person who, at age 45, became so convinced by his own research, that he took up running. In his early 80s, he had more than

---

55 Bortz, 1991.

150 marathons and ultramarathons to his credit. By this time, he was an avid ultramarathon runner and preparing for a 100 mile run, up and over the Sierra Nevada from Lake Tahoe to Auburn, California. Dr Paffenbarger was involved with a long-term study about health, known as the Harvard Study.

Eric Olsen was a student who wanted to be a pilot. He was covering the 100 mile race for a running magazine and wanted to interview Paff, who eventually agreed. Although they did not get on famously at the start, they eventually struck up a relationship and went on to write their book *LifeFit* in 1996. Their book advocates the importance of physical activity and maintaining muscle mass for the pursuit of successful ageing. Dr Paffenbarger maintained that 'it is never too late to take up an active life'.[56] Dr Paffenbarger helps us to understand the importance of exercise on the ageing process. He describes how we can change our ageing curves depending on our commitment to exercise and a healthy diet.

Dr Paffenbarger created his own **Blueprint for Successful Ageing** when he became convinced by his own research and discovered running.

Ruth Heidrich – *A cancer survivor who became an athlete*

Ruth Heidrich was diagnosed with breast cancer at 47. A surgeon removed a tumour the size of a golf ball from her breast and subsequent tests confirmed that it was malignant. When she asked her oncologist why a fit and healthy person who had taken good care of herself had cancer, the reply was simply,

56 Paffenbarger & Olsen, 1996.

we don't know. After a battle with an aggressive breast cancer, and a radical mastectomy, it was unclear whether the cancer had spread beyond the breast to bone, liver, lung or brain – the most common places where this form of cancer metastasises. Fortunately, the cancer had not spread, and Heidrich recovered.

Rather than treating this life-threatening experience as a reason to withdraw from society, it became, as she describes, a very strong motivator. Heidrich refused chemotherapy and radiation and adopted a plant-based diet, largely removing all animal protein. She also set about getting fit. Already a marathon runner, she went on to compete in six ironwomans and win 67 marathons including Boston and New York. Heidrich became a committed vegan and wrote the well-recognised 2005 book, *Senior Fitness: The Diet and Exercise Program for Maximum Health and Longevity*. Heidrich is a role model and provides a classic example of how disease can become a distinct motivator to commence or continue exercising while pursuing a healthy diet.

Heidrich created her own **Blueprint for Successful Ageing** by beating cancer, becoming a gold medal-winning athlete and author, and eating a plant-based diet.

• • •

In summary, attitude is an essential part of who we are. If we are positive, we will find it easier to achieve better outcomes, whereas if we are negative, we will find excuses for not achieving our goals. If we have a negative attitude, we are more likely to be affected by stereotyping and ageism. If we are positive, we can pass on our positivity to others. A compliment is always better than a criticism and a compliment will be more appreciated, and leave both parties feeling better about themselves. Whether we get out of bed in the morning to go training or put it off for another day because we don't feel like it, is a function of attitude. Remember, *if you think you can, or if you think you can't, you are probably right!*

In the next chapter we will look at whether you have a positive or negative attitude to ageing, take a quiz to figure out which of the three ageing curves you might belong to, and look at opportunities for improvement.

Before you read on, pause and consider these two questions:

1. **Find a role model you admire, someone who has a blueprint for successful ageing that impresses you. When you feel like being inactive or eating poorly, ask yourself – what would my role model do?**

2. **What can you do today that will display your positive attitude?**

CHAPTER 5: HOW POSITIVE IS YOUR ATTITUDE?

A positive attitude to ageing

In this chapter we will test your positivity and your approach to successful ageing. As I have said, a positive attitude is a catalyst for getting out of bed in the morning. It helps you commit to exercise, a nutritious diet, and it provides you with the confidence to maintain your social networks. As we observed in the previous chapter, people with a positive attitude are also better able to solve problems as they are continually looking at other options to find a solution.

During the research for my PhD, I was continually impressed by the positive attitude exuded by the Elders that I interviewed. Remember, these people had an average age of 86, and a couple were centenarians. Although all of the Elders had retained a positive attitude, most of them had experienced some form of emotional or physical setback and been able to overcome it. Those with a positive attitude are better equipped to deal with the challenges that regularly confront them, and they can remain optimistic about the outcome. These people are often referred to as 'the glass half full group'.

A positive attitude is essential to having the best quality of life.

A negative attitude to ageing

In contrast, those with a negative attitude to life will be eternal pessimists, anticipating that every problem will result in disaster. A negative attitude to ageing or older people is referred to as ageism and the term was widely accredited to Dr Robert N. Butler in 1969. Dr Butler (1927-2010) was an American physician, gerontologist, psychiatrist and author, who suggested that older people are perceived as inactive, forgetful, intellectually rigid and ready to be superseded by a younger model. He referred to this as a process of systematic stereotyping or discrimination against people who are old.[57] He won the Pulitzer Prize for General Non-Fiction in 1976 for his book *Why Survive? Being Old in America.*

Sadly, the type of ideology that equates ageing with deterioration robs hope from everyone at all stages of life. Similarly, the negative terms used to perpetuate stereotypes against older people include geezer, old fogey, old mate and old goat. *Healthy at 100* author John Robbins – who helped popularise the link between diet and physical health and who advocated for whole foods and a plant-based diet for ethical, environmental and health reasons – discusses what he calls the 'still syndrome'.[58] This is a series of questions that the young adopt when they are speaking with the old.

For example, are you still working? Are you still driving?

---

57 Butler, R.N. (1969). Age-ism: Another form of bigotry. *The Gerontologist, 9(4)*, 243–246.
58 Robbins, 2006.

Are you still managing on your own? These comments are demeaning, create a feeling of hopelessness and can result in an older person withdrawing from society. Ageism is a prejudice against a group that even the young will inevitably join if they live long enough. One of the key drivers for ageism or devaluing old age is said to be due to a fear of what lies in store for us!

Our doctors and many health professionals also contribute to this stereotyping and ageism. I am certain that older readers will have been advised by at least one of their doctors, 'what do you expect, you're not getting any younger'. Or in my case, 'stop pushing yourself!' The way we respond to these stereotypes can influence our own potential to pursue an active lifestyle in our senior years. It can also determine the way we treat others. Stereotyping is unnecessary and hurtful; it robs older people of their confidence and can affect their self-perception.

When we take these negative comments personally, we start believing what these naysayers are spruiking. In contrast the Abkhazians and Vilcabambians celebrate ageing, and their elderly people are held in great respect. The older the person, the greater the respect. During my PhD, I faced heavy criticism for researching health and ageing, given I am a town planner. Thankfully, with some positive encouragement from my supervisors, I persevered. There were still numerous occasions when I thought I would never get there.

Most people have an unrealistic appreciation of their own commitment to looking after their mind, body and overall health. Basic recommended levels of physical activity are inadequate and misleading. Walking is better than nothing, but not enough to combat the overweight, loss of muscle mass and fitness problems. Also, descriptions of healthy food leave most of the population confused about whether they are making correct decisions about what they eat. The following section will help you to analyse your commitment to a healthy and successful lifestyle.

Know your ageing curve

Taking an analysis of our own lifestyle can help us assess how quickly we will decline. In the theory of ageing, Australians can fit within one of the three ageing curves. These ageing curves can indicate a person's biological age and are summarised from levels 1 to 3, as follows:

Level 1 Successful ageing curve

A person on the successful ageing curve is fully committed to a healthy and active lifestyle, and is pursuing plenty of exercise, a plant-based diet, and the other key successful ageing components.

Level 2 Optimistic ageing curve

A person on the optimistic ageing curve is generally committed to a healthy and active lifestyle and has some appreciation of some successful ageing components.

Level 3 Typical ageing curve

A person on the typical ageing curve thinks ageing and decrepitude are inevitable. They may also be unaware or uninterested in the successful ageing components. Some may have genetic health problems.

Which of these three ageing curves do you feel best describes your understanding and commitment to a healthy lifestyle? As a guide for identifying which category might best describe your lifestyle, consider this quick quiz. This is not a medical quiz and should not be considered to be a substitute for medical advice.

Quiz

1. Do you undertake moderate to vigorous levels of exercise for more than 60 minutes at least 6 days a week?

Yes	No

Note: For people aged 65 years and over, the recommendation is at least 30 minutes of moderate intensity physical activity on most, preferably all, days.[59] Countless studies have shown that this is a bare minimum, and greater benefits can result from an increased commitment. My research concludes that 60 minutes, six days a week, is optimum.

2. Do you try to include physical activity in your daily life?

Yes	No

Note: Opportunities for physical activity are available everywhere in our daily lives. For example, using stairs rather than lifts or elevators, walking rather than driving to shops and facilities, including a walk or bike ride in the journey to work or place of entertainment, and walking at every opportunity. Also, standing rather than sitting for long periods at work, standing up every 30 minutes if you are watching TV or sitting on the lounge, stretching regularly or using stretch bands to help mobility.

3. Does your understanding of nutrition assist you in pursuing a healthy intake of a variety of vegetables and fruit?

Yes	No

---

59 Australian Government. (2025). *Physical activity and exercise guidelines for all Australians.* https://www.health.gov.au/topics/physical-activity-and-exercise/physical-activity-and-exercise-guidelines-for-all-australians

Note: Most Australians don't consume enough vegetables and fruit, and consume too much refined food containing added salt and sugar. While almost all vegetables can be consumed in abundant quantities, with an emphasis on variety, fruit has high levels of fructose, which is in fact sugar and can increase sugar consumption. The recommended intake from the Australian Dietary Guidelines is two pieces of fruit and five or six serves of vegetables a day for males and females aged 15 years and over.

4. Do you enjoy none, one, two or three glasses of alcohol daily and have the willpower to stop then?

Yes	No

Note: While some people argue any alcohol is bad for you, observations of long-lived people have shown social and health benefits from moderate consumption of alcohol.

5. Are you within the healthy weight and waist parameters with a BMI that is normal for your age group?

Yes	No

Note: As we age, many of us gain weight and lose muscle mass. Frequently, muscle may be replaced by fat. Maintaining muscle mass and waist dimensions are highly desirable health parameters. Body Mass Index (BMI) can assist in identifying healthy weight, overweight or obese parameters.

6. Have you been able to avoid the need for medication for high blood pressure, cholesterol, excess sugar, type 2 diabetes or other biomedical risk factors?

Yes	No

Note: If you have been able to avoid medication for biomedical risk factors, you are in the minority in our ageing population – well done!

7. Do you visit your local GP, dentist or specialist on an annual basis to have a health check, skin check, your teeth checked, a blood test, stress test or other assessments to determine if you have any potential health risks?

Yes	No

Note: Having annual check-ups are essential preventative health measures that we should all undertake. These visits and/or tests can provide early warning signs of preventable biomedical risk factors that can require much greater intervention if left unchecked.

8. When you visit your GP, dentist or specialist, do you go prepared with a series of questions, ask them to explain your blood test results, make careful notes of their comments, and carefully file these comments and any test results to enable you to refer to them as necessary?

Yes	No

Note: When you visit your health experts, prepare a list of questions and record the answers. This is a very important step in your prevention of future illness. Being as informed as possible will allow you to make better decisions.

9. Does your diet minimise your consumption of fast food, sugar, sugary drinks, salt and refined foods? Do you adhere to the 80:20 Rule (eating healthy and nutritious foods 80% of the time)?

Yes	No

Note: Do you consume a balanced diet and minimise refined food and takeaways to about 20% of your diet? Our changing society has made it easy and cost effective to consume increasingly high levels of high density, fast and refined food. Most of this fast food has high levels of salt and sugar to stimulate our tastebuds and ensure that we eat more than we need.

10. Have you managed to avoid disease (cancer or heart disease) or been able to fully recover from that type of life-threatening experience?

Yes	No

Note: Lifestyle has been found to be a major contributing factor to cancer and heart disease. If you have been able to avoid cancer or heart disease, or been able to fully recover, you probably have had, or now have, a healthy lifestyle and become more conscious about the things you do on a daily basis.

Results

If you have answered yes to nine out of 10 questions and ticked yes to questions 1, 3, 4, 5, 6, 9 and 10 then it is likely that you are on the successful ageing curve. Well done, you are in good shape!

If you have answered yes to seven or more of the 10 questions, and ticked yes to questions 1, 3, 5, 6, 9 and 10, then it is likely that you are on the optimistic ageing curve, which means you are conscious about your daily pursuits but could make changes to your lifestyle to enhance your health and wellbeing.

If you have answered yes to six or less of the above questions, then you are likely to be on the typical ageing curve. It's also likely that you need to be convinced to make a change. Even the smallest change in your daily routine could improve your health and wellbeing and reduce the potential biomedical risks you are facing and the likely disease, disability and/or early death that you will experience. The more we expose our bodies to the key behavioural risk factors, the more we are exposed to downstream biomedical risk factors.

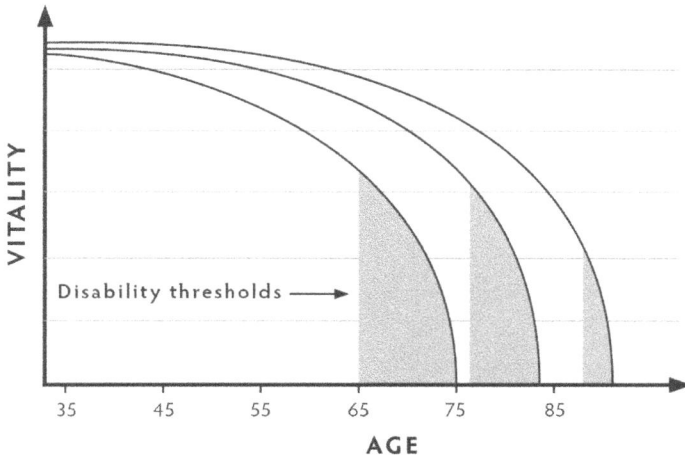

Figure 5.1: The three ageing curves: Usual, Optimistic and Successful and the Disability Threshold. Source: Author's compilation.

Room for improvement

A dear and departed close friend of mine would respond to questions about his health by saying, 'it is the largest room in my house for improvement'. Unfortunately, in his case this proved to be true, and his passing at age 68 was very sad for all those who knew this sharp and effervescent personality. Regardless of which of the three categories you self-assessed your current lifestyle to fall within, there is always room for improvement.

You may never have any desire to be in the successful ageing curve – to be an obsessive or committed person who carefully programs their physical activity and is conscious about the food they consume. However, if you are on the typical ageing curve, with a number of behavioural risk factors, then there are some very compelling reasons why you should take action to improve your lifestyle, reduce biomedical risk factors and lower the likelihood of disability and disease.

If you are sedentary, improving physical wellbeing comes slowly, but it is a vital first step.[60] Reducing the risk of heart disease must be a prime motivation, as coronary heart disease is the top killer of men in Australia and the second-highest cause of death in women (Alzheimer's is first for men and second for women). However, there are obvious biomarkers, such as having a healthy BMI, having the recommended waist measurement (under 94cm for men and 80cm for women), and healthy blood pressure, just to mention a few. Countless studies have validated the benefits of engaging or re-engaging in exercise and consuming a better diet. Start walking, join a gym, eliminate sugar, salt and refined foods, and you will be moving yourself from the typical ageing curve to the optimistic one. Unless we are genetically compromised or have been subject to irreversible disease or major trauma, most of us can pursue this second option.

It's often said that a person has been 'unlucky' if they develop cancer or heart disease – and sometimes that's true, particularly at a young age. But more often than not, these life-threatening conditions can be traced back to lifestyle choices.

Everyone is ageing. If you are not ageing, you are dead. However, the good news is that most of us can control our biological ageing and slow down the onset of disease, disability and death. I would like my last decade on this earth to be as active and pleasurable as possible. Wouldn't you?

---

60 Paffenbarger & Olsen, 1996.

In summary, if you have self-assessed your ageing curve as 'typical', don't be depressed. The room for improvement is extensive and potentially untapped. Even small improvements will yield benefits, and if you continue to introduce positive changes, you will notice an enhancement to your health and general wellbeing.

If you have categorised your ageing curve as 'optimistic', then you are doing reasonably well. Depending on your age, improving your lifestyle might assist in further deferring your entry into the medication or disability zone. You are probably the most fortunate if you fall within this category, as you are committed enough to not want to fall into the 'typical' category and enthusiastic enough to want to improve.

If you have categorised yourself in the 'successful' ageing curve category, you have probably found that a number of people think you are not only obsessive but really quite mad! Many people simply do not understand that 'successful ageing' people get a buzz from high intensity exercise and healthy food. It is simply incomprehensible for someone in the typical ageing category to appreciate that it can be very enjoyable exercising to exhaustion and then celebrating by tucking into a simple vegetable stir-fry or a crisp green apple. However, if you have assessed yourself as in the successful ageing curve category, you have a duty to share the secret of your **blueprint for successful ageing**, with as many people as possible.

In the next chapter we will examine the vital importance of nutrition, the various diets out there (I also road-test some of the more popular and well-known ones), my own diet and preferred foods, drinks and supplements, my 10 nutritional rules, and the importance of avoiding unhealthy processed foods.

Before you read on, pause and consider these two questions:

1. Are you happy with how you scored in the quiz? Which ageing curve are you on right now? What do you see as your strengths and weaknesses?
2. What ageing curve do you aspire to in 12 months' time? What things are you prepared to change?

CHAPTER 6: NUTRITION – YOU ARE WHAT YOU EAT!

Why is food important?

Remember when you were young and your mother or father would tell you, 'You are what you eat', as they were trying to encourage you to eat your vegetables? Well, unsurprisingly, your parents were right! A more accurate comment is 'your mood is reflected by what you have eaten'. You may have observed an obstreperous child, only to find they have consumed large amounts of sugar. Heather Morgan, a US health coach, reminds us that 'every time we eat or drink, we are either feeding disease or fighting it!'

Most people don't make the connection between the food they eat and the quality of their health. When I interviewed my then GP, he freely admitted that he had not received any training on nutrition. I was amazed. He was a great GP and had years of experience; yet he was flying blind when it came to our body's most important fuel. Hippocrates, the father of medicine (460-357 BC), is credited with saying, 'he who does not know food, how can he understand the diseases of man?' The overwhelming body of research concludes that the food and nutrients we consume largely determines our wellbeing, our level of inflammation, the efficiency of our immune system, and our susceptibility to disease. Over millennia our food consumption habits have changed dramatically. This chapter considers some of those changes, over the past 200 years, and how our diet has evolved from the hunters and gatherers, through the meat and three veg era of the 1950s and '60s to our current multicultural/Australian diet, which is high in salt, sugar and refined foods.

Hunter and gatherer diet

For thousands of years, the First Nations people in Australia were fishermen, as well as hunters and gatherers. If they lived near the coast, seafood was a major source of food. Away from the coast, wild animals, plants and berries were consumed, depending on what was available. Following colonisation, the early settlers, who didn't have the knowledge or skills of the First Nations people, adopted European techniques of farming animals and cultivating crops. Two different food cultures prevailed: the Indigenous or natural culture, living off the land and water; and the European culture, farming animals and growing crops. Regardless of the culture, food had to be farmed or hunted, and exercise was an essential part of the day from when our predecessors woke until they retired, ensuring calories were burnt off and few were overweight.

The interwar diet

There are some interesting facts about the interwar diet. Hygiene in food shops became much better, fresh fruit was available all year round, and the milk supply was much cleaner. This all changed with the declaration of World War II in 1939. During the war, food rationing of bacon, butter, sugar, meat, tea, cooking fat, cheese, eggs and milk resulted in people being much slimmer, with few people being overweight. In particular, there was a low level of obesity. There was less food to go around for the majority of the population, and many people could have been described as being lean and hungry. This was an involuntary form of food restriction or limiting portion size.

These observations were also made in Europe when the Germans invaded towns and cities, and confiscated poultry, sheep and cattle for the German armies. This necessitated a dietary change for many of the villagers across Europe. This pattern is consistent with research that shows that eating less food, in particular less meat and more grains, vegetables and nuts, resulted in fewer overweight or obese people.

Meat and three veg

As a baby boomer living in a small flat in Bondi, I was raised on what was then considered to be an Australian diet of 'meat and three veg'. Almost every night we would have chops or sausages with three vegetables and that began my love affair with mash potatoes that prevails today. Chicken was relatively expensive and therefore a rarity. On Friday evenings, we had the luxury of fish and chips from the local fish shop. Sunday was always a roast for lunch, and you would never miss this weekly extravaganza.

Fundamentally, this was a reasonably healthy diet. The meat was invariably grilled, and my mother would always steam the vegetables, in a pressure cooker, to retain nutrients. Also, we consumed very little processed food. In Bondi, there were very few takeaway outlets and even fewer restaurants. The few milk bars and hamburger shops were the focal point for young people to gather and socialise. I recall seeing very few overweight people, and this observation is supported by statistics.

The hamburgers in the '60s and '70s were far more nutritious than the Big Macs we know today. A hamburger with 'the works' might have included lettuce, tomato, beetroot, an egg, and real mincemeat in a bun. The homemade patty had relatively low levels of sugar and salt, which is in contrast to the high levels contained in today's fast food.

The evolution of the Australian diet

In the 1960s and '70s, Australia began its journey to becoming a multicultural nation. Our European diet was influenced by the numerous new cultures arriving on our shores. The First Nations diet had been usurped by European influences and only prevailed in central and outback Australia. Greece, Italy, Lebanon, China and Japan, then later Vietnam, Turkey and India, began to influence our food preferences. However, the American influence, due to the rise of a global culture, has been the most dominant and, arguably, the most detrimental to our health.

McDonald's and Coca-Cola set the trend for refined foods and sugary drinks in North America in the 1970s, and this trend soon spread around the world. Australia closely follows the eating trends of North America, particularly refined, high density, unhealthy, sugary foods, which are low in any nutritional value. McDonald's, Hungry Jack's, KFC and Krispy Kreme are just a few of the sugar-laden habits we have had foisted upon us, by US multinationals.

Recently my wife and I cooked a tofu pasta (gluten free) and veggie stir-fry, with a glass of red wine, which was amazing and very nutritious. However, the normal daily Western diet is seldom this nutritious. On a daily basis, most Australians eat highly refined processed foods and sugary drinks, which could easily contain 40-50 teaspoons of sugar. This is more than four times the recommended level in Australia, with WHO guidelines recommending only about 12 teaspoons a day. I have discussed our problems with sugar consumption in Chapter 9. Canadian cancer researcher and author of numerous books on health, Dr Richard Beliveau, describes the Western diet as follows: 'With all I have learnt over these years of research, if I were asked to design a diet today that promoted the development of cancer to the maximum, I could not improve on the current Western diet.'[61]

Although he was describing the North American diet, the Australian diet follows close behind. Also, Australians are becoming increasingly lazy, with the introduction of home deliveries from all of the fast food providers. If we don't call in or grab a takeaway on the way home, we can order one to be delivered, right to our doorstep. Ordering or grabbing a takeaway meal from a fast food outlet foregoes some of the old-fashioned habits of standing around in the kitchen and cooking a wholesome and nutritious meal, while socialising

---

61 Beliveau quoted in Servan-Schreiber, D. (2010). *AntiCancer: A new way of life*. Penguin.

with friends and family, which is a very pleasant experience. Misleading packaging on refined food and sugary drinks is the most disturbing (see Chapter 9).

Food manufacturers put such massive amounts of refined sugar in foods for a simple reason – to stimulate appetite.[62] People whose appetites are stimulated eat more food, and in turn consume excessive amounts of sugar. They also buy more! This is a particularly disturbing observation. Not only is the Western diet contributing to our population of overweight and obese people, a considerable amount of research confirms that it is also contributing to the risk of various cancers. Research by geneticist and cancer researcher Professor Thomas Seyfried suggests that cancer is a metabolic disease that feeds on sugar, and that the high levels in our diet make us more prone to the disease. There is considerable evidence to support the reduction or elimination of sugar from our diet.

Types of Australian diets

Although I prefer the terms food and nutrition to describe what we consume on a daily basis, the word diet has been adopted by the food industry to describe our sustenance. There are countless books that make unsubstantiated claims about various diets that you are encouraged to follow, in order to achieve health and longevity. A snapshot of some recent popular diets includes Atkins, Ketogenic, Paleo, the CSIRO Total Wellbeing Diet, 5:2, Blood Type, Anti-cancer, Pescatarian, Mediterranean, Sardinian, Harvard, Pritikin, Vegetarian and Vegan. In descending order,

---

62 Robbins, 2006.

these diets move from meat-based to plant-based. The authors spruiking each of the above diets make compelling arguments why their diet is superior. After researching most of these diets, my conclusion is that there is no one diet that is suitable for everyone. For myself, I have found that the Mediterranean diet has been the most helpful.

As part of my research, I 'test drove' many of these diets to see if they were appropriate for my metabolism. You can read more about my findings below.

Atkins

The high animal protein Atkins diet did not work for me, as I am accustomed to fresh fruit and a lot of vegetables, and a concentration of meat was not good for my system.

Of course, many people swear by low carbohydrate keto diets like Atkins. But while there are claims that red meat offers a good source of protein and can assist in losing weight, there is also research that has found that excessive consumption of animal protein can be carcinogenic.

The Australian Cancer Council recommends people consume moderate amounts of unprocessed (or fresh) lean red meat. A moderate amount of meat is no more than 455g cooked red meat (equal to about 700g raw meat) per week. This could be a small 65g serve of cooked meat each day or two serves (130g) three times a week. Americans have always consumed a considerable amount of red meat. However, the newly revised set of Dietary Guidelines for Americans (DGA) recommends limiting consumption of animal proteins.[63] It also recommends that beans, peas and lentils be reassigned from the 'vegetable foods group' to the 'protein foods group'. And also, that this group be listed as first protein options, followed by nuts, seeds, and soy products, then by seafood, and finally by meats, poultry and eggs as last options. Processed meat, with the unknown levels of preservatives, carries the strongest carcinogenic warnings. This could be a new direction for America, if they follow the guidelines.

The Australian Dietary Guidelines state:[64]

- Enjoy a wide variety of nutritious foods from the five food groups every day.
- These five food groups are:
  - o fruit and vegetables;
  - o potatoes, bread, rice, pasta and other starchy carbohydrates;
  - o beans, pulses, fish, eggs, meat and other proteins;
  - o dairy and alternatives; and
  - o oils and spreads.
- Drink plenty of water.
- Limit the amount of food you eat that contains saturated fat, added salt, added sugars and alcohol.
- Protect, support and promote breastfeeding.
- Be food safety aware.

---

63 U.S. Department of Agriculture and U.S. Department of Health and Human Services. (2025). *Dietary guidelines for Americans, 2025-2030.* https://www.dietaryguidelines.gov.
64 Australian dietary guidelines. www.eatforhealth.gov.au

In the end, while Atkins may work for some, the evidence suggests that a diet high in red meat and low in plant-based foods is neither sustainable nor optimal for long-term health. Indeed, Dr Atkins died of heart disease at age 72 – not a great endorsement for his life's work.

Ketogenic

The ketogenic diet, often called the keto diet, is a very low carbohydrate, high-fat diet that forces the body to burn fat for energy instead of glucose (sugar). This metabolic state, called ketosis, occurs when the body produces ketones from fat breakdown, which can be used for energy. The diet is characterised by very low carbohydrate intake and replacing it with high fat, with moderate protein intake. While I have not tried this diet, much of it would work for me. However, losing my muesli and mash potatoes would be a problem. On a serious note, a friend of mine, who declined radical surgery and chemotherapy for breast cancer, credits the keto diet and creating a metabolic state of ketosis for eliminating her cancer.

Paleo and Blood Type

The Paleo and Blood Type diets have interesting attributes. I had difficulty with the Paleo diet, with the exclusion of cereal and legumes, and an encouragement to eat large amounts of fruit.[65] Rolled oats and other grains play an important part of

---

65 See for example Cordain, L. (2010). *The paleo diet revised*. Harper Collins.

my breakfast.[66] I do consume fruit, but I believe an abundance of fruit (fructose) increases sugar levels.

The Blood Type diet maintains you should eat a diet most suited to your blood type.[67] Its creator, American physician Dr Peter D'Adamo, maintains that your blood type determines your susceptibility to illness, which foods you should eat, and how you should exercise. For example, Type O is the original blood group of our earliest inhabitants, while the Type A and B groups are said to have evolved as the population migrated to hotter climates in different parts of the world. As I am Type O, I am a carnivore, which I certainly was in my younger days, regularly consuming a steak that would cover the whole plate. These days, red meat plays a much smaller role in my weekly meals, and therefore the Blood Type diet dropped off my list. With a reduced consumption of meat, my digestion is improved, and my bowel movements are more regular.

Pritikin, Vegetarian, Vegan and 5:2

The Pritikin diet was developed by Nathan Pritikin, an American engineer and nutrition pioneer, after he reversed his own heart disease through lifestyle changes in the 1970s. Rich in fruits, vegetables, whole grains and low in fat, it is supported by research for its heart health benefits, although some find it overly

---

66 Oats are not gluten free and not suitable for people with Coeliac disease but are generally well-tolerated by people with gluten intolerance. See: https://coeliac.org.au/

67 D'Adamo, P. (1998) *The eat right diet: A simple guide to eating right.* Century.

restrictive. I found the Pritikin, Vegetarian and Vegan diets caused me to lose weight, which some might say is an advantage. I thought the Pritikin diet was close to the Mediterranean diet with an emphasis on fruit, vegetables, wheat, dairy, and lean protein, that includes fish and red meat. I choose not to have dairy, and I have to avoid wheat, which contains gluten. I could survive on a modified Pritikin diet.

Vegetarian and Vegan diets left me hungry an hour after I ate; obviously I was not including enough protein. My niece, who is a vegan, would argue I didn't consume the correct food, and she is probably correct. Her vegan recipes are excellent, but above my level of skill.

Interestingly, she has recently been diagnosed with osteoporosis, which can be a result of a number of factors, not the least of which can be a lack of protein. This is my real concern with both of these diets. At my age, it's a continual battle to consume enough protein to maintain my muscle mass.

I also found that the 5:2 diet (five days of routine eating and then limited calories for two) was not enough to sustain my calorific needs, given my current level of exercise. For people who are overweight, I can see the distinct advantage of reducing how many calories you consume in a day or week, which is the feature of the 5:2 diet. However, I have the reverse problem, trying to keep weight on! My wife and many of my friends say that is a nice problem to have.

Pescatarian, Mediterranean, Sardinian and Harvard diets

Accordingly, my shortlist was the Pescatarian, Mediterranean, Sardinian and Harvard diets. All of these diets have unlimited fresh fruit and plenty of vegetables. I float between these four diets. I could be a pescatarian and have fish every day. The Sardinian diet has an emphasis on bread and cheese, which did cause me some concern and there seemed to be fewer fresh vegetables, so this diet is a struggle for me. I found the Harvard diet was very precise, although perhaps somewhat overregulated. The Harvard diet has a Healthy Eating Plate as the focus and divides food into four categories with a proportion for each. Wholegrains and healthy protein were 25% each; with vegetables and fruit making up the other half of the plate. Obviously, there is much more detail about each of the food items in each group. I could survive on this diet.

I settled on the Mediterranean diet as it seems to have a greater reliance on seasonal fresh produce to the almost total exclusion of refined foods (see Figure 6.1).

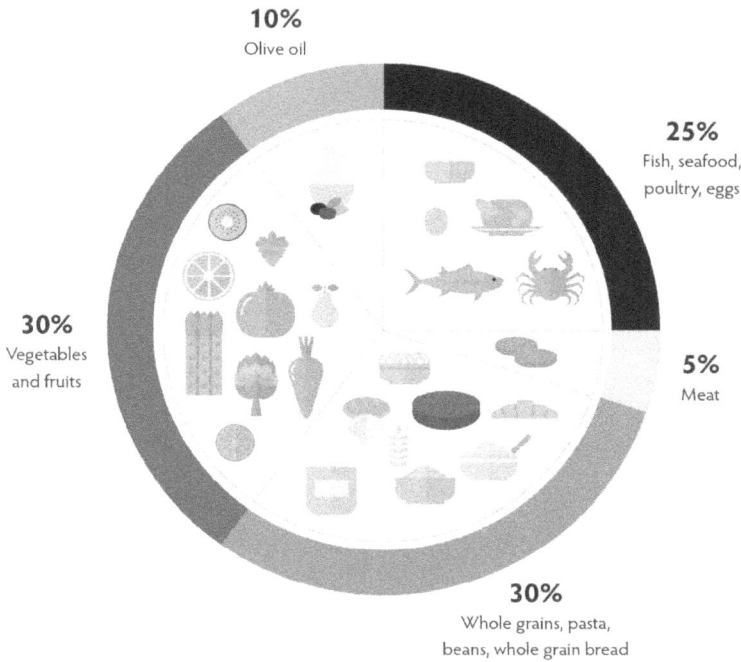

Figure 6.1: An example of a Mediterranean Diet. Source: Modified image from Shutterstock.

My top pick – the Mediterranean diet

There are different interpretations of the Mediterranean diet, depending on which part of the world you live. My preference is a plant-based interpretation with plenty of fresh vegetables, nuts, seeds, olive oil and a limited amount of fruit, with three servings of fish (preferably oily) three times a week. To satisfy my passions I can readily incorporate my pescatarian and carnivore cravings into my Mediterranean diet without compromising the nutritional benefits. The other benefit for me is that it's relatively easy to identify and eliminate gluten, which is my Achilles heel. In my view, it is the unknown additives included in refined foods that is causing many of the health, obesity, diabetes and cancer problems we have today.

Dr Robert H. Lustig is Professor Emeritus of Pediatrics, Division of Endocrinology at the University of California, San Francisco. He has fostered a global discussion of metabolic health and nutrition, exposing some of the leading myths that underlie the current pandemic of diet-related disease. In his 2021 book, *Metabolical*, Dr Lustig argues you only need to know two precepts: first, protect the liver. Second, feed the gut. Only eat real food that doesn't contain toxins or other poisons. This is a solid recommendation, one that I support. Remember Heather Morgan's caution, 'Every time we eat or drink, we are either feeding disease or fighting it!'

The Mayo Clinic identifies the ultra-processed foods and beverages with the most potential to do damage to our health.[68] These ultra-processed options tend to contain:

- five or more added ingredients;
- added sugar, salt, oils, fats, stabilisers and preservatives;
- additives that imitate the flavour, colour or texture of less processed foods; and
- ingredients not found in nature, such as high fructose corn syrup.

---

68 Mayo Clinic Press. *Key ingredients to avoid in ultra-processed foods.* https://mcpress.mayoclinic.org/nutrition-fitness/key-ingredients-to-avoid-in-ultra-processed-foods/

They're also defined by what they don't contain. These ready-to-eat products are often so processed that vegetables, grains and other unprocessed foods are either barely present or absent.

A critical benefit of the Mediterranean diet over the current Western diet is the absence of refined food and the presence of fresh seasonal fruit and vegetables with the addition of plenty of nuts. In my opinion, refined sugar and sugar generally is our arch enemy, and we should avoid it at all costs, except where it occurs naturally in foods. In contrast, the health benefits of the Mediterranean diet are well documented, with evidence to support lower cholesterol and blood pressure, while reducing the risk of diabetes and cancer. Importantly, its other health claims include increasing our health span and a greater potential for longevity.

The 2024 book, *My Mediterranean Life*, by Australian nutritionist Sarah Di Lorenzo, has a number of Mediterranean recipes that I am working through, and which I would highly recommend.

My 10 nutritional rules

We all have different nutritional needs, and it is not my intention, or my role, to tell you what to consume. However, the rules I have arrived at, and try to live by, after 80 years on this planet, are as follows:

1. Start the day with a hot squeezed lemon juice to cleanse/activate.
2. Remember the 80:20 Rule, and try and do the right thing 80% of the time.

3. Eat slowly, chew thoroughly, pause regularly and stop when 80% full.
4. Eat the rainbow in vegetables and two or three pieces of fruit per day.
5. Consume between 80-130g of protein throughout the day.
6. Eat a variety of nuts, some dried fruits and a spoonful of olive oil.
7. Avoid salt and sugar wherever possible.
8. Avoid refined food, unless the contents clearly articulate the benefits.
9. Avoid deep fried and energy-dense food.
10. Avoid the unhealthy fats.

It is also critical to remain hydrated. Almost all of us are dehydrated for part or all of the day. Keep drinking water throughout the day.

While these rules work for me, they may not work for you and at the end of the day it is your body, and you should know, or you should learn, how to look after it. Some people are insulin resistant or may have other dietary requirements that may render my diet totally unsuitable. We all have our own needs, problems and peculiarities and you should get your own advice before following any of my habits.

My preferred foods

I also have a number of 'go to' foods which I try to include in my weekly diet. I don't profess to be a nutritionist; however, during my time on this planet, I have made plenty of mistakes and hopefully learnt from them. My preferred foods and my reason for selecting them are included here. There are many claims about the cancer-protective qualities of the following foods, which is beyond my expertise. What I can say is that my health is much better, and my immune system is stronger, when I am consuming a broad spectrum of the following foods and drinks.

Fruits

Food	Key Nutrients	Benefits
Blueberries & blackberries	Antioxidants, polyphenols	Boost memory, improve blood flow, lower blood pressure, anti-inflammatory
Bananas (best slightly green)	Carbohydrates, tryptophan, Vitamin B6	Sustained energy, mood support, gut health
Avocados	Monounsaturated fats, potassium, Vitamins B6, E, K	Supports heart health, glowing skin, healthy cholesterol
Other fruits (2–3 per day)	Varies	Fibre, vitamins, hydration, natural sweetness

Vegetables

Food	Key Nutrients	Benefits
Leafy greens (broccoli, spinach, kale)	Vitamins C & E, antioxidants	Immune support, anti-inflammatory, protects cells
Root vegetables (carrots, beets, sweet potatoes)	Beta carotene, fibre	Eye health, stable energy, antioxidant support
Greens (peas, beans, sprouts, bok choy, lettuce)	Vitamins A, C, K, folate	Bone health, immunity, digestive support
Mushrooms	Antioxidants	Immune support, may lower inflammation

Legumes, Grains & Soy

Food	Key Nutrients	Benefits
Legumes (beans, chickpeas, lentils)	Fibre, plant protein	Helps lower blood pressure, stabilises blood sugar
Rolled oats & grains (excluding wheat)	Soluble fibre	Supports healthy cholesterol, balances blood sugar
Soy & tofu	Protein, copper, calcium, selenium, phosphorus	Plant-based protein, bone health, hormone balance

Protein (Animal)

Food	Key Nutrients	Benefits
Ora king salmon & sardines	Omega-3 fatty acids, calcium	Heart and brain health, bone density

Meat (chicken, fillet steak, lamb cutlets)	Protein, iron, B vitamins	Muscle maintenance, energy
Eggs	Protein, Vitamin B	Supports lean muscle, satiety, brain health
Yoghurt	Probiotics, calcium	Gut health, digestion, bone strength

Healthy Fats & Oils

Food	Key Nutrients	Benefits
Olive oil (1 tbsp)	Polyphenols, antioxidants	Heart-healthy, anti-inflammatory, good substitute for butter
Nuts & seeds	Protein, Vitamin E, Omega-3	Supports immune system, healthy fats, satiety
Avocados (also listed under fruits)	Healthy fats	Cardiovascular and skin benefits

Herbs, Spices & Extras

Food	Key Nutrients	Benefits
Garlic	Allicin, antioxidants	Lowers blood pressure and cholesterol
Ginger	Anti-inflammatory compounds	Aids digestion, reduces inflammation
Dark chocolate (in moderation)	Iron, magnesium, antioxidants	Reduces inflammation, supports mood

Drinks

Drink	Type / Notes	Recommended Quantity	Benefits
Water	Filtered where possible, with Hydralyte after training	8-10 glasses per day	Excellent daily hydration & electrolyte balance
Coffee	Strong soy flat white	1-2 cups per day	Energy boost, antioxidants (in moderation)
Tea	Green tea	1-2 cups per day	Antioxidants, supports metabolism
Red Wine	Shiraz	2 glasses per day (except Mondays)	Polyphenols, heart health (in moderation)
Beer	Tooheys Old	1 stubby per day (except Mondays), perhaps an extra 1 or 2 on the weekend	Relaxation, social enjoyment (in moderation)

Studies show coffee and tea contains an abundance of health-protective substances like flavonoids that are thought to protect cells from damage as well as keep inflammation in check. Caffeine and coffee have been found to reduce the risk of Alzheimer's, Parkinson's and other degenerative brain diseases. Caffeine consumption is also associated with several other benefits.[69]

---

69 Cho, S., Kim, K.M., & Chu, M.K. (2024). Coffee consumption and migraine: A population-based study. *Scientific reports*, *14(1)*, 6007. https://doi.org/10.1038/s41598-024-56728-5

By altering levels of brain chemicals involved in mood, caffeine consumption may reduce risk of depression. However, sweetened soft drinks and energy drinks come loaded with added sugar and few, if any, nutrients. Still other drinks combine the health-promoting substances from coffee or tea with hefty amounts of added sugar and fat. Some of these blended coffees and teas contain more calories, sugar and fat than most frosted and cream-filled donuts. Beware of products claiming to be healthy.

My preferred supplements

There are many publications about the benefits or otherwise of supplements and it is difficult to find any that are truly objective and without skin in the game. As it is a multi-billion-dollar business, there are many to choose from.

I have taken a variety of vitamins over the years, and I have decided those that help to boost my immune system work for me. Mind you, that doesn't mean they are suited for you or anyone else. Also, there are some I take every day and others every second day. I found taking all of these vitamins every day was too much for my system and made me feel lethargic. I also have at least one day a week vitamin free. Recently, I have started taking Ginkgo Biloba and I have observed some improvements in my recall of previous events. I have also started taking Creatine monohydrate, which is said to help produce adenosine triphosphate (ATP) – a source of energy that your cells use when you exercise. I am now taking both daily.

Daily	Vitamin C, fish oil, magnesium, CoQ10, ginkgo biloba, and creatine
Every second day	Vitamin B12, Vitamin D3, Vitamin K2

Allergies and food intolerances

Our current Australian diet includes high levels of energy-dense food that contains excessive levels of sugar, salt and unhealthy fats that make our bodies work harder and become more vulnerable to insulin resistance, allergies and food intolerances. Insulin is a hormone produced by the pancreas, which regulates blood glucose levels by promoting glucose storage in fat cells, inhibiting lipid breakdown and, stimulating protein synthesis. It also helps sugar move from your blood into your cells.

Insulin resistance occurs when cells in your muscles, fat and liver don't respond to insulin as they should. This is also known as impaired insulin sensitivity and can lead to diabetes. Insulin is essential for life and regulating blood glucose (sugar) levels.

Many children are born with allergies that they grow out of in adolescence. As mentioned earlier, I was born with an inordinate number of food allergies and, most importantly, an allergy to the lifesaving drug at that time, penicillin. I did experience one allergic reaction in later life, when I inadvertently consumed jellyfish as part of a Chinese banquet. I became itchy in minutes, went into anaphylactic shock and ended up in hospital. I didn't know I was allergic to jellyfish until that time. While I grew out of all the above allergies, except jellyfish and penicillin, by choice I now largely avoid dairy, pork, salt, sugar and by necessity any food containing gluten.

If our stomach has an overload of sugars, salts and refined foods, we can also end up with various types of food intolerances. People with these food intolerances or sensitivities can't break down certain foods in the gut. Insulin resistance, discussed elsewhere, can lead to a variety of metabolic problems.

The difference between a food intolerance and a food allergy is quite important. An intolerance causes symptoms like an upset stomach, rashes and problems with the digestive tract from consumption of what might be only a small sample of this disagreeable food. Importantly, it is not life-threatening. I experience these symptoms when I incautiously consume gluten. On the other hand, an allergy activates the immune system, which releases antibodies (proteins) called immunoglobulin E to fight the threat. Allergic reactions can include hives, swelling, shortness of breath, wheezing, and anaphylaxis. They can be life-threatening.

Although my diet largely excludes dairy, salt, sugar and almost all refined foods, I developed an undiagnosable reaction to the consumption of some foods that plagued me for several years. Bread, pies, pastries and pasta were the main offenders, and I loved pasta and crusty Italian bread. Visits to doctors, dermatologists, gastroenterologists and dietitians – and undertaking numerous tests – failed to diagnose my problem.

My reaction after consuming the offending food begins with a rash on the left arm, which then manifests itself on the chest, buttocks and groin, before affecting my digestive system and bowel movements. For many years I had no idea how to treat this disorder as it would result in me being overwhelmingly tired, with an inability to concentrate.

Out of sheer frustration, I pursued an unsupervised, unsophisticated series of food elimination tests and landed on gluten as the potential source or main contributing factor to my problem. Out of the 14 most common symptoms for gluten intolerance, I had at least eight of them. These symptoms included skin problems, feeling tired, headaches, bloating, diarrhoea and constipation. Not a pleasant topic, but a critical piece of self-diagnosis.

Since laying at least part of the blame on gluten and gluten intolerance, the good news is that I did not have Coeliac disease, and it was something that I could manage with some major dietary adjustments. We tried tracing events back to the start of my problem, and the only link was a trip to Moscow when Vicki and I got food poisoning. And no, we could not prove it was linked to Mr Putin!

What is gluten? Gluten is a family of proteins found in grains like wheat, rye, spelt, barley, and many other grains. Gluten is formed when proteins glutenin and gliadin, present in flour, are combined with water, and is readily available in flour, dairy products, starch breads, pasta and noodles. Although gluten lacks any nutritional benefits, it is useful for binding bread, pasta and many other processed foods. Not surprisingly, we are seeing an increasing number of Australians who are gluten intolerant and there is a growing number of products that are gluten free. While my wife thinks pursuing a gluten free diet is a pain in the butt, it won't hurt you and, in fact, you are likely to feel better.

Avoiding unhealthy processed food

If you are living in a city, town or urban area, it is extremely difficult to avoid consuming processed foods. It is even more difficult to determine what is good for you and what is killing you. We are continuously misled by marketing and packaging, and our inadequate food regulations allow manufacturers to be totally disingenuous to a naïve consumer. However, there is a new sheriff in town, which is an app called Yuka, that I have road-tested and it is awesome. This app can measure almost all refined food with a barcode, give it a health rating out of 100 and tell you whether it is excellent, good, poor, or bad for you. It also provides a breakdown of the positive and negative attributes of the product. The positives might include fibre and protein content, while negatives might include the number of additives, and the level of sugar, calories and sodium.

I was suitably shocked to find out that the apparently healthy gluten free fig biscuits that I quite enjoyed had a rating of 24 out of 100 and were described as bad. My old favourite Vegemite had a rating of 48 out of 100 and was rated poor. A number of other items that I purchased from the so-called healthy food shelves in the supermarket also rated extremely badly. The good news is that gluten free Weet-Bix, olive oil, blackberries, blueberries, tofu and yoghurt – an essential part of my daily regime – rated 90+ and were identified as excellent. Since discovering the Yuka app, I have carried out an audit of our pantry and, to my wife's chagrin, thrown out a whole pile of unhealthy food stuffs. I would suggest you test the app yourself on your own pantry and see if it helps you to make healthier choices next time you are at the supermarket.

My daily diet

We all have our likes and dislikes which determine our preferences. Although my diet varies slightly each day, I endeavour to apply the 80:20 Rule and not be too naughty on the 20% days. However, my diet does seem to work for me and generally speaking it includes the following:

Meal	Description
Brekkie	• Glass of water • Large bowl of homemade muesli with rolled oats, rice bran, prunes, figs, raisins, LSA (linseed, sunflower seeds, almond meal), black chia seeds, organic brown flaxseeds, desiccated coconut, and a high proportion of roasted nuts (almonds, Brazil nuts, cashews, hazelnuts, pecans, walnuts, macadamia nuts) • Served with blackberries and blueberries, sliced banana, soy milk, and yoghurt • Optional: slice of gluten free toast with olive oil plus avocado or an egg, or both • Coffee
Alternative (2 days/ week)	• Hot brekkie: two poached eggs (or scrambled), spinach, avocado, gluten free toast • Coffee (Known as 'Gary's Brekkie' at the golf club)
Lunch	• Glass of water • Mixed salad or veggie wrap with a protein feature (e.g. smoked salmon, tofu, or sardines)

Dinner	• Glass of water • Main: fish, tofu, pasta or meat • Accompanied by stir-fry or microwaved or steamed vegetables (at least four varieties) • Optional: scoop of gluten free light yoghurt with fruit (preferably apricots) and a piece of dark chocolate • Glass or two of red wine (preferably shiraz)
Notes	• Olive oil used in place of butter • Avoid salt and sugar
Snacks	• Nuts and a piece of fruit • Possibly a second coffee

In summary, diet and nutrition are very much a personal thing. It may be that more or less meat works for you; alternatively, you may be healthier with a vegetarian or vegan diet. The facts are, our diets have evolved over the past 50 years and not necessarily for the better. Most Australians have an unhealthy diet, which is defined as inadequate amounts of fruit and vegetables and an overconsumption of refined foods that contain excessive amounts of salt, sugar and unhealthy fats. Also, our food and our eating habits encourage overeating.

The research, and in particular observations of the longest-lived people, would suggest that a plant-based Mediterranean diet has stood the test of time, and we can learn from the Japanese by stopping eating when we are 80% full. (Remember: *hara hachi bu*).

In the next chapter we will look at why exercise is the most important thing in our lives, various myths about exercise, what type of exercise is best for you, guidelines to getting started, successful exercise case studies, and the importance of your own personal exercise program (PEP).

Before you read on, pause and consider these two questions:

1. **How would you rate your diet? Do you consume enough vegetables and fruit; and do you limit the amount of sugary drinks, fast food and processed food?**
2. **What are three things you could do to improve your diet? Write them down. Can you do them?**

CHAPTER 7: WHY EXERCISE IS THE MOST IMPORTANT THING IN OUR LIFE

History and myths about exercise

Exercise for the purpose of training to increase strength, speed and endurance can be traced back to ancient Greece around 600 BC. Greek and Spartan soldiers were among the first to engage in exercise, such as lifting heavy rocks and doing construction work to increase muscle strength, running long distances to increase speed and endurance, and competing in wrestling matches to refine fighting skills.

The tale upon which the modern Olympic marathon rests is the mythic run of Pheidippides from Marathon to Athens. He was a professional messenger and, in 490BC, is supposed to have brought a message from the plains of Marathon, where the Greek Army had just won a crucial battle against the invading Persian Army of General Datis. After the battle, in which he may have taken part, he was dispatched to Athens to deliver the news: 'Rejoice, we are victorious.' He is thought to have said this, then dropped dead with exhaustion.

Subsequently, exercise for the purpose of training led the military to the idea of competition, and then to the first Olympics in ancient Greece. Socrates (470-399 BC), credited as the founder of

Western philosophy, was also an advocate for exercise. He argued that each person has a responsibility to develop their physical capabilities to their fullest potential. He believed that physical strength, alongside mental strength, was crucial for overall development and wellbeing. According to a quote attributed to him by Xenophon in his *Memorabilia*, Socrates argued: 'No man has the right to be an amateur in the matter of physical training. It is a shame for a man to grow old without seeing the beauty and strength of which his body is capable.'

The fact is that over many thousands of years humans have relied on movement to escape predators, sow crops, or simply to travel from one location to another. Our bodies are designed for movement and the more frequently we pursue a variety of movements, the better our bodies respond to the ravages of ageing. I discussed my evolving exercise passion in Chapter 1. I argue that exercise is the closest thing to a panacea for successful ageing; add a healthy diet and you have the almost complete package.

Defining physical activity and exercise

The WHO defines physical activity as 'any bodily movements produced by skeletal muscles that require energy expenditure and produces progressive health benefits'.[70] The term 'physical activity' should not be confused with 'exercise', which is a subcategory of physical activity that is planned, structured, repetitive, and aims to improve or maintain physical fitness.

---

70 WHO. *Physical activity.* https://www.who.int/southeastasia/health-topics

Regardless of definition, if we have a higher level of fitness and mobility, there is less stress on our body and heart when we are walking, moving or performing difficult tasks; we function more efficiently. In contrast, for a person with a low level of fitness, even the simplest movements are an effort. Our appreciation of exercise has evolved with the advance of science in sport and the development of sophisticated training programs to achieve specific goals.

Duration and type

The Harvard School of Medicine recommends at least 150 minutes of moderate-intensity activity or at least 75 minutes of vigorous-intensity activity and at least two strength training sessions (even 10 to 15 minutes is good) per week for adults.[71]

The Australian Government also advises two strength sessions per week. It recommends 2.5 to 5 hours of moderate intensity physical activity such as a brisk walk, golf, mowing the lawn or swimming; or 1.25 to 2.5 hours of vigorous intensity physical activity such as jogging, aerobics, fast cycling, soccer or netball – each week for adults aged 18-64.[72] For people aged 65+, the Australian Government says at least 30 minutes of moderate intensity physical activity on most, preferably all, days is recommended. It's my view that older people should get 60 minutes of exercise six days a week.

---

71 Harvard Health Publishing. (2025). *A three-pronged approach to exercise.* https://www.health.harvard.edu
72 Physical activity and exercise guidelines for all Australians. https://www.health.gov.au/topics/physical-activity-and-exercise/physical-activity-and-exercise-guidelines-for-all-australians

I suggest there are three levels of physical exercise:

- Light exercise: you don't feel like you're exerting yourself.
- Moderate exercise: you can talk comfortably but not sing.
- Intense exercise: you can say a few words, but not full sentences. Within the guidelines, one minute of intense activity is roughly equivalent to two minutes of moderate activity.

Although we are training for the marathon of life and not an Olympic event, there are some compelling arguments that we need to include vigorous or intense exercise as an essential part of our training program. My opinion is the Darwinian theory still applies in present-day society – the fitter we are, the better our chances of a long and healthy life. Also, as strength and muscle mass is declining as we age, I believe a 70+ person has to do more exercise than a 40+ person to retain strength.

Type of exercise

Exercise is safe for almost everyone – even people with chronic disease and disabilities. Also, different types of exercise have complementary benefits:

- Aerobic exercise, like walking, running, or cycling, improves cardiovascular health. It involves movement of the large muscles of the body for sustained periods of time.
- Muscle-strengthening exercise, like resistance training with elastic bands or weightlifting, improves muscle strength, endurance, power and muscle mass.

- Bone-strengthening exercise, like running, playing basketball, resistance training or jumping rope, improves bone health and strength.
- Balance exercise, like walking backwards, standing on one leg, yoga and tai chi, can reduce the risk of falls.
- High Intensity Interval Training (HIIT) is training at near maximum effort. As this form of exercise has found to be particularly beneficial to older people, I have included some research about it below.
- Multi-component exercise, like running, surfing, dancing, golf or playing tennis, includes at least two of the above types of activity.

Which exercise is best for you?

The type of exercise which is best for you is subject to a diverse array of opinion. Walking is the most popular form of exercise for people over 60 years of age. While walking is great and most people can do it, walking doesn't help to retain bone density or to stave off osteoporosis. You can enhance the level of cardio fitness from walking if you pursue a fast pace or incorporate hills and stairs.

All of the research acknowledges the benefits of maintaining muscle mass and how increasing the muscle-to-fat ratio can increase your aerobic capacity and the health of your cardiovascular system. Muscle mass also helps to retain your metabolic rate, which helps you to burn fat.

Strength training regularly helps preserve lean muscle tissue and can even rebuild some that has been lost already. Weight training has also been shown to help fight osteoporosis. Studies by University of Sydney geriatrician Professor Maria Fiatarone Singh showed that even 80- and 90-year-olds can improve strength and muscle mass.[73]

Also, to achieve the maximum benefit from my suggested 60 minutes of exercise six days a week, it needs to be personalised and carefully structured.

Intensity of exercise

There is considerable debate about the intensity of exercise that should be pursued. Although health professionals agree that exercise is of considerable benefit to everyone, opinions are divided over whether greater benefit is obtained from some, more or less vigorous levels of exercise. As health professionals are often conservative, a few that I have interviewed felt that a low to moderate level of exercise should be recommended.

My personally documented observations over 60 years have found that the more exercise I do, the better I feel and the fitter I am. Sounds crazy for an 80-year-old! A relevant and recent meta-analysis of one million individuals produced some

---

73 Fiatarone, M.A., Marks, E.C., Ryan, N.D., Meredith, C.N., Lipsitz, L.A., & Evans, W.J. (1990). High-intensity strength training in nonagenarians. Effects on skeletal muscle. *Journal of the American Medical Association*, 263(22), 3029–3034. See also, Fiatarone, M.A., O'Neill, E.F., Ryan, N.D., Clements, K.M., Solares, G.R., Nelson, M.E., Roberts, S.B., Kehayias, J.J., Lipsitz, L.A., & Evans, W.J. (1994). Exercise training and nutritional supplementation for physical frailty in very elderly people. *The New England Journal of Medicine*, 330(25), 1769–1775. https://doi.org/10.1056/NEJM199406233302501

interesting conclusions. The study found that low volumes of exercise are associated with large risk reductions for all causes of cardiovascular mortality.[74] Increasing volumes of exercise yielded additional health benefits, but there was an absolute decrease in mortality risk, for every doubling of exercise volume. Vigorous intensity exercise was associated with the lowest mortality risk. The study concluded: a little is good, more is better, and vigorous is best.

Framework

Exercise has changed from an activity we did on weekends to an essential part of health and wellbeing for many of us. Unfortunately, there is a large proportion of the population who do not appreciate the joy and benefits that accrue from regular exercise. My observations from a lifetime of exercise provide the context for my commitment and recommendations in the following sections.

Shortly after I joined the North Bondi Surf Club in 1964, I began recording my daily exercise, the results, and any injuries or illnesses I may have incurred. These records enable me to evaluate which programs worked best for me and modify my training to improve results. My objective is to provide you with a blueprint for your daily exercise, and this blueprint will be the most important commitment you can make for your body. Regardless of the intensity you pursue, exercise is good for both

---

74 Eijsvogels, T.M.H. & Maessen, M.F.H. (2017). Exercise for coronary heart disease patients: Little is good, more is better, vigorous is best. *Journal of the American College of Cardiology, 70*(14), 1701–1703. https://doi: 10.1016/j.jacc.2017.08.016

mind and body at any age. As they say, in the classics, 'what is good for the heart is good for the head'.

My lifetime exercise philosophy, which I outline in Chapter 1, is confirmed by the findings from the study mentioned previously: little is good, more is better, vigorous is best. And surely, we all want the best for our bodies. I recently attended a club reunion, where I have been a long-time member, and almost all of those in attendance, who were somewhere near my age, were pursuing very little exercise. Most were overweight and many were quite unwell. Sadly, a few had passed prior to our reunion, and a few have passed since. We will all pass eventually; however, my long-term goal is to die as young as possible (biologically), and as old as possible (chronologically).

Let's consider the benefits of exercise, getting started, enjoying the journey, establishing goals, and developing your program. Hopefully by the time you finish this chapter, you will be convinced that strength and aerobic exercise and a few other pursuits will enhance your sense of wellbeing as you age. You can also have a lot of fun in the process.

The benefits of exercise

Exercise is the most important commitment you can make to your day. It activates your mind, stimulates muscles, maintains bone density and helps to stave off osteoporosis. As our late friend Professor Julius Sumner Miller would say, why is it so? As we observed, if we are sedentary as we chronologically age, we lose muscle mass and strength from age 35. Imagine losing almost half your strength by the time you are 80! You go on holiday and cannot pick up your suitcase. I am in my 80th year and I am lifting heavier weights now than I ever have before and I have improved my grip strength.

In contrast, a sedentary 80-year-old male, having lost 40% or more of his strength and muscle mass, is likely to have a slower metabolism, an increase in fat stores, sarcopenia (muscle wasting), loss of bone density and perhaps osteoarthritis. One in three people over 65 will have a fall each year and may go to hospital or die, primarily, due to frailty resulting from a loss of strength and muscle mass. This would be a major reduction in the activities you could enjoy daily or at worst the downward spiral where you never recover. This does not need to be your fate!

Every day we need to resist the temptation to be sedentary. Exercise is also your most important asset in the war against obesity, heart disease, cancer, dementia, and type 2 diabetes. It can change your outlook from negative to positive, change your mood from unhappy to happy, and change outcomes from failure to success. I have regularly found that a run, walk, swim, ski paddle, gym workout or round of golf in the morning sets me up for the day. We all need to keep moving, because if we are standing still, we are effectively going backwards as we age.

Finally, it's my belief that if our exercise level is at a relatively high intensity and we progressively overload the muscles at subsequent training sessions, our white cells are tricked into the growth phenomenon rather than death, decay and dying. I am trying to convince you that exercise will help keep you in the growth and regeneration mode of life, until you ultimately die. This is one of the pathways to lowering your biological age.

Getting started guidelines

If you are a regular trainer, the following section may be well-known to you. However, it may also act as a refresher. The first step before starting an exercise program is a full medical check and blood test. Ensuring that there are not any underlying health issues is an important prerequisite before changing your lifestyle. When you begin or recommence training, it is important to diarise your baseline fitness or benchmark. These markers will become incredibly important as you move forward and measure your improvement.

Some of the biomedical measurements are blood pressure, cholesterol LDL (low-density lipoproteins), HDL (high-density lipoprotein), triglycerides, iron and mercury, uric acid and rested heartbeat. You might also check your VO2 max. If you are already on medication for any of these biomarkers, discuss any risks with your GP, but don't be persuaded not to exercise. Ensure that you get these results from your GP and learn to understand them – don't just take your doctor's word for it that you are okay for your age or too old to do anything. The key physical health markers I suggest you monitor are weight, waist, BMI, rested heartbeat and blood pressure, grip strength, leg strength and walking up two flights of stairs (without puffing). Going forward I suggest that you measure your weight daily at the same time each day (best first thing in the day) and write it down and measure your waist once a week. If you have a smartwatch, you can check many of these markers when you choose.

It is also desirable to measure body fat to muscle ratio and your visceral fat (belly fat). This measurement can readily be obtained from a Dexa scan. I have one of these scans annually; it is a great way to monitor body fat and visceral fat. Visceral fat is a type of body fat that's stored within the abdominal cavity and can cause health problems immediately. Visceral fat increases insulin resistance, which can raise blood pressure and lead to type 2 diabetes, various cancers and heart problems. On a positive note, you will be surprised at the rush of enthusiasm you will enjoy from losing a few kilos or some visceral fat from around your waist, in your quest for successful ageing.

Having fun and enjoying the journey

An important aspect of developing a regular exercise program is to make it enjoyable. Firstly, it has to be fun to keep you doing it! If it's a run or walk, select an attractive environment, whether it's natural in a bushland or park setting, coastal with headlands, beaches and waterways, or a built environment with some attractive open space, landscaping or pedestrian activity that provides highlights, preferably with no cars.

Secondly, the selection of your gym is of critical importance. The gym needs to have state-of-the-art, safe equipment, excellent instructors and there needs to be a high standard of hygiene. If users are not wiping down the equipment before and after usage it is not the right culture for you. The people using the gym will also tell you a lot about the management and the culture. Are they friendly, welcoming and helpful? Are they people you will look forward to seeing on a regular basis?

It may be that running and gyms are not for you; don't stress, there are many other options. If you are a walker, that is fine, except you will need to up the ante, to provide some resistance or weight bearing during your walks. You can include stairs in your walk, increasing the number of stairs as you get fitter; or you can walk with a backpack with weights in it, increasing the weights gradually over time. This will help maintain bone density and improve cardio fitness. Pilates offers opportunities to build strength and gain flexibility, with Pilates mat, and reformer. The mat exercises are on the floor, and the reformer is on a specially designed machine.

Yoga is also excellent for strength and flexibility and balance. You will need classes and an instructor for Pilates and yoga. Swimming and cycling are great for your heart and cardio fitness, but they won't help to maintain muscle mass and bone density. Other activities to consider include rowing, ski or canoe paddling, rock climbing, tennis and pickleball; the options are endless. As a ski paddler for over 50 years, it is the ultimate escapism, out in the ocean paddling through waves or on the harbour, dodging the ferries; it is great strength and cardio exercise, and a lot of fun. Try any or all of the options, but when you pick your preferred activities, pick and stick.

Thirdly, make your exercise sessions fun and enjoyable. Maybe have a small celebration at the end of your training session. It is sometimes good to have a different group of friends for each activity. My wife, Vicki, has two groups of girlfriends who she trains with – the walkers and the gym goers – and they always have a mandatory coffee after their training session. Every other day Vicki and one girlfriend sit down with a crossword when they have their coffee. Catching up for a coffee after exercise strengthens social bonds, builds a sense of community, and turns movement into a shared ritual that supports both physical and emotional wellbeing. These after-training pleasures are also the rewards for getting out of bed and exercising.

Establishing goals

It is important to have short-, medium- and long-term goals to focus your exercise. Then you can develop an exercise structure to achieve your goals. These goals are critical to measure outcomes and develop the package of what I label your personal exercise program (PEP). It is not simply a matter of rocking up to the gym for a few weights or going for a bike ride. With a PEP in your pocket, or on your phone, you have thought about the short-, medium- and long-term goals that you want to achieve.

You not only have goals, but you also have an *ikigai*; your long-term goal becomes your purpose for exercise, or at least one of them. The first realisation is that this is a lifetime commitment, not something you do for a few weeks or months. If you're not in there for the long haul you might need a softer approach. So how might this PEP work? For example, you might decide your goals are as follows:

- Short-term: lose 5kg, exercise 5 days/week for 30 minutes, walk and weights.
- Medium-term: lose 10kg, exercise 5 days/week for 60 minutes, walk, weights and swim.

- Long-term: lose 15kg, exercise 6 days/week for 60 minutes, walk the City2Surf.

My approach is to decide on your long-term goal first, then you know where you want to be. Then, determine the short- and medium-term goals that will get you there! I thought about this long and hard and this is the way I approach my goal setting!

It is useful to record your sessions on your phone or in a notebook – wherever you will enjoy observing your improvements. I record my sessions in a weekly Outlook program, and it is the first and last thing I do on the computer each day. When you achieve your long-term goal, in say, 12 to 18 months, establish a new goal and adjust your medium- and short-term goals accordingly. You may consider adopting this goal-oriented approach for other aspects of your life, as it helps to strengthen your purpose (your *ikigai*) for being here.

Case studies

Let's consider three hypothetical case studies using three 60-year-old males in varying physical condition. These hypothetical men have set their goals, and the following exercise component is only indicative. I have selected age 60 as it is a critical period in ageing, when you set yourself up for your next 30-40 years. This decade, when many are retiring, is also known as the slippery 60s, where some start the downhill slide.

Let's look at the indicative goals for these three hypothetical case studies.

Case Study 1: *60-year-old man on a typical ageing curve*

Profile	
A 60-year-old male currently on the typical ageing curve trajectory. Previously trained but now in poor condition. He is 110kg (20kg overweight), qualifies as obese, is pre-diabetic, with high blood pressure and high cholesterol. On multiple forms of medication.	
Goal	**Prescription**
Long-term goal (12 months)	Achieve optimistic ageing curve trajectory. Reduce weight from original 110kg to 90kg (-20kg), reduce waist size to <90cm, lower blood pressure and cholesterol, avoid diabetes, reduce medication, and mitigate other risk factors.
Short-term goals (3 months)	Reduce weight from 110 to 105kg (5kg) and waist measurement to 94cm. Strength goals: 3x10 push-ups, 3x5 assisted chin-ups, 3x5 deadlifts at 45kg, 3x6 curls at 5kg, 200 abs, 1-minute plank. Improve VO2 max: walk 5km or swim 400m. NB: Goals are indicative for beginners, adjust accordingly if more experienced.
Medium-term goals (3-9 months)	Continue weight loss to 95kg. Strength goals: 3x20 push-ups, 3x8 assisted chin-ups, 3x5 deadlifts at 50kg, 3x8 curls at 6kg, 200 abs, 2-minute plank. Improve VO2 max: complete City2Surf in <100 minutes or participate in North Bondi 1km or 2km swim. All goals should be tailored with a trainer.

Case Study 2: *60-year-old man on an optimistic ageing curve*

Profile	
A 60-year-old male currently on the optimistic ageing curve trajectory. He is 90kg (10kg overweight), slightly high blood pressure and cholesterol, some risk factors, and on two forms of medication.	
Goal	*Prescription*
Long-term goal (lifetime pursuit)	Move from optimistic ageing curve to successful ageing curve. Reduce weight from 90kg to 80kg and create his own blueprint for successful ageing.
Short-term goals (3 months)	Reduce weight to 85kg and reduce waist measurement to <94cm. Strength targets: 2x20 push-ups, 2x5 chin-ups, 3x5 deadlifts at 50kg, 200 abs. NB: These goals are indicative for less active individuals; targets should be set to challenge, not discourage.

Medium-term goals (3-9 months)	Run the City2Surf in under 80 minutes or complete the North Bondi 1km or 2km swim. Reduce weight from 85kg to 80kg and reduce waist measurement <90 cm. Strength goals: 3x20 push-ups, 3x8 chin-ups, 300 abs, 2-minute plank, 1x30 seconds obliques each side. Improve VO2 max: 8x400m on 2:15 min, run 10km in 60 minutes.

This hypothetical male might also see a few improvements in his biomarkers: increased muscle mass, a slight lowering of his blood pressure or lowering cholesterol. Continuing to monitor the improvements in biomarkers will give him a physical and mental lift. Implicit in these outcomes might be cutting back or eliminating his medication. Some doctors may say this is irresponsible or impossible. In fact, in most cases, it is achievable.

Case Study 3: *60-year-old man on a successful ageing curve*

Profile	
A 60-year-old male on the successful ageing curve trajectory, aiming to maintain his fitness level.	
Goal	*Prescription*
Long-term goal (12 months)	Remain on successful ageing curve and follow own blueprint for successful ageing. May also wish to set personal challenges to sustain motivation and progression.
Short-term goals (3 months)	Focus on structured programs designed to support medium- and long-term goals. No weight issues, no risk factors, and not on medication. Goals should offer challenge and continuity.
Medium-term goals (3-9 months)	Run City2Surf in under 60 minutes or win age group in North Bondi 1km or 2km swim. May set additional power/weight goals to enhance strength and preserve muscle mass.

The case studies are based on male body weight and measurements, but the principles and exercises apply equally to women. In my world, men and women perform the same exercises and most of the time, women do them better.

I regularly set myself short-, medium- and long-term goals, which help me to focus, define or redefine my PEP, which I will discuss now.

Personal exercise program (PEP)

Having a PEP is the semi-final step in completing your blueprint for successful ageing. It can also become an important part of your *ikigai*. It is not possible to provide an exercise program for everyone in this chapter as we all have different goals and different levels of fitness. However, having established your goals, you or your trainer will be in a good position to develop your PEP.

Look at your PEP as a lifetime journey, where you are continually changing gear to deal with the topography; there will be numerous highs and a few speed humps. You will also need to continually review your goals. Then, learn to sit back, relax and enjoy your exercise program. You have heard the term, if you enjoy your job, you will never work a day in your life! Well, exercise is the same; if you can develop a passion for your PEP, you will be looking forward to your next workout and be buzzing at the end of each session. You won't need any drugs, you can get your highs from a good workout in the gym, a hard swim, a good run, or a solid Pilates session. You can also feel secure in the knowledge that you have earned your brekkie, lunch, a cocktail, or dinner. The additional good news is the benefits from your intense workout goes on for hours after you have finished your session. Your body is recovering, your metabolism is up, and you are still burning energy and fat.

Your proposed PEP is to achieve the short-, medium- and long-term goals you have designed for yourself, or with a trainer. I highly recommend working with a trainer, as they will set a program you can build on, as well keep you motivated and attentive to technique. Also, the motivational power of competition – having a clear goal, objective and shared benchmark, be it a fun run or ultramarathon – can't be overstated. It drives consistency, sharpens focus, and delivers a powerful sense of achievement even on the days you don't feel like showing up.

If you are starting off, you will need to build up by increasing training sessions from 30 minutes to 60 minutes and from five sessions to six sessions a week. I have included seven sessions of approximately 60 minutes in the duration in the PEP, which is based on my program. I recommend six sessions and a rest day for you, and they need to be planned and programmed. There might also be a few gratuitous stretching, balance or flexibility activities, that are over and above the six sessions. I say gratuitous as they are not a substitute for the core training program.

The 60-minute duration workout in the gym is based on a ladder format and the need to warm-up and cool down. If you are doing Pilates or yoga classes it will likely follow a similar format, warm-up and cool down with the effort in the middle and about an hour duration. The start of each workout is the bottom of the ladder: from light to moderate, building to intense; hold the intensity for 30 to 40 minutes; then move down the ladder to moderate; then light. For instructors and those who train regularly, it may seem like common sense. However, having watched numerous people train for different sports over a lifetime, most do not maximise their training efforts. Here are some important tips when you are using the gym or training generally.

Tips

- Breathing correctly is of prime importance. Breathe in through the nose on recovery and out through the mouth on the effort. Regulate your breathing to develop a rhythm or flow.
- Posture and technique should be constantly in your mind. Mirrors or an instructor are useful to ensure your stance and efforts are technically correct.
- Balance is essential when you lift weights or perform any exercise.
- Ensure your weight is equally distributed on both feet, knees, hips and arms.
- With weights, I prefer to have a quick effort (exhale), and a slow (three second) recovery (inhale).
- Try leaving your phone in your locker when you go to the gym.
- Work one-on-one with a skilled trainer – the benefit will outweigh the expense.
- Work towards a competitive goal – register for a fun run or half marathon and lock the date into your diary.

Light, moderate and intense zone workouts

A gymnasium workout starts with a light training zone with light efforts – in other words, you are telling your body to get ready to move to the next level. This might be, say, five minutes on a strider or pulleys, or the rowing machine. Then, in the moderate zone, once your heart rate is at about 50-60% of maximum, you move into your first, lighter weight set. For example, a warm-up bench press might be with 2x7.5kg dumbbells, and the pull-ups are with one 12.5kg dumbbell, alternating to each arm.

Next, we move into the intense/vigorous training zone. As you build strength in this zone, you will see your heart rate go between 60-80% of maximum for between 30-40 minutes. Initially, in this zone, use a weight you can easily lift seven times, gradually increasing the weight. Ideally, as you get stronger you increase the weight until, in subsequent sessions, you are struggling or failing to lift your last repetition in each set. As one exercise is pushing you, the other is pulling you; this results in you getting cumulative, yet positive/negative weight loading on a similar muscle group. This type of lifting is often referred to as super sets. To get maximum benefit, you need to keep moving during this routine with a different exercise or a stretch – don't sit down and play with your phone while you recover! Some brief stretching of chest and arms will be helpful. An advanced super set routine might include six groups of two or three exercises in each group, with four sets and seven repetitions. Start with the larger muscle groups, chest, back and quads, then move to the smaller groups, arms and legs (see below).

An example super set routine

Group 1	Bench press, pull-ups + shrugs. Recovery: stretch arms and chest.
Group 2	Quad + hammie machines. Recovery: 10 squats with 2x5kg weights.
Group 3	Leg press machine + balance on one leg with a weight in one hand, swap.
Group 4	Curls and triceps + step-up on a bench with weights
Group 5	Adductors (both machines, push + pull). Pause at the end of the effort.
Group 6	Ski machine (1 min hard) and some abs. Include obliques + planks.

For beginners and intermediate trainers, an easier option to stay in the intense zone, and build up to super sets, is to use different muscle groups. For example, use arms, then legs, moving from one muscle group to another. As we are looking for muscle mass and strength, we need more weight and less repetitions (reps). I have suggested four sets, first one as a warm-up, the next three sets near max weight with seven reps. If you are doing some maximum weights on dead lifts or leg press, you need recovery time, but not on your phone. Use the recovery time to work on your balance, perhaps on one leg moving a weight from one hand to another as mentioned above or stretch the worked-on muscle group.

To finish the workout, move back down the ladder to the moderate/light zone. I recommend 5-10 minutes on abdominals and planks + stretching, and flexibility.

An example of my typical strengthen/weight session is included in Table 1 below. As a warning, my routine may be seen by some as excessive or extreme, which is probably true. Stretching is important after a weight routine as weights shorten the muscles, and as we age it becomes more important to lengthen them. I also like to do another light stretching routine before bed.

Table 1: Typical strength/weights session		
Intensity	Exercise	Comment
Light warm-up	Strider (5 minutes) Pulleys (5 minutes, 20 reps each)	Warm-up all muscle groups
Moderate	Bench press + pull-ups Shrugs, leg press machine	First set – use lighter weights to get muscles ready for heavier weights
Vigorous	Bench press + pull-ups. Shrugs, leg press machine, squats, balance on foam with weights	Second to fourth sets – perform at near max. Arms recover doing legs, legs recover doing arms
Vigorous	Wall squat with weight Hammies + quads (1 min)	First set lighter, next three sets at near max
Vigorous	Curls + tris + step-ups on box with weights	First set lighter, next three sets at near max. Arms recover while legs are working, cardio effort is maintained
Moderate	Adductors both machines + balance	One set warm-up, three sets of push and pull (7 reps super sets)

Light	Abs (300), planks 2 mins, obliques + stretching	Warm down

Note: Guidelines for Table 1 Weight Session

Sets: 4 sets including 1 warm-up set

Weights: First set 60% max. last 3 sets with weight 80-90% max

Repetitions: First set 10 warm-up; 7 last 3 sets

Heart rate: Light 20-50% of maximum HR

Medium 50-60% of maximum HR

Vigorous 60-80% of maximum HR

(Depending on age)

Maximum heart rate is 220 minus your age.

Table 2 is my Seven Day PEP, for each day with a comments column. I review my PEP regularly and have a break from routine every month.

Table 2: My typical weekly program		
Day	**Exercise type**	**Comment**
Monday	Recovery day: Ab Lab: stretch + Pilates + abs Light swim or run	No efforts above 70% Stretch/Pilates/abs with my regular squad
Tuesday	Swim 2km with squad, followed by Pilates session Swim, maybe replaced by a run	Any form of cardio + abs + Pilates

Wednesday	Golf 18 holes + swim 1km	Fun day of golf + swim
Thursday	Strength workout: AM heavy weights + abs; PM soft sand run	See Table 1 Heavy weight morning, cardio afternoon
Friday	Cardio: Swim 2km with squad + abs; golf 9 holes	Any form of cardio + abs Swim, stretch + abs
Saturday	AM HIIT Session + abs; PM golf	Make time for other exercises, e.g. ski paddle
Sunday	Cardio: AM swim 2km + stretch PM hit golf balls	Make time for other exercises, e.g. pickleball

You will observe from the above, my PEP in Table 2 is for seven days. This PEP is for someone who is no longer working full time. It is difficult to pursue my PEP if you are working full-time. Also, you need to design your PEP to meet your short-, medium- and long-term goals. While I recommend everyone pursue six days, I feel I am missing something if I don't have a commitment every day. Perhaps this is one of my obsessive-compulsive problems, that I will discuss in a later chapter. A photo of my Ab Lab and a swim squad are below.

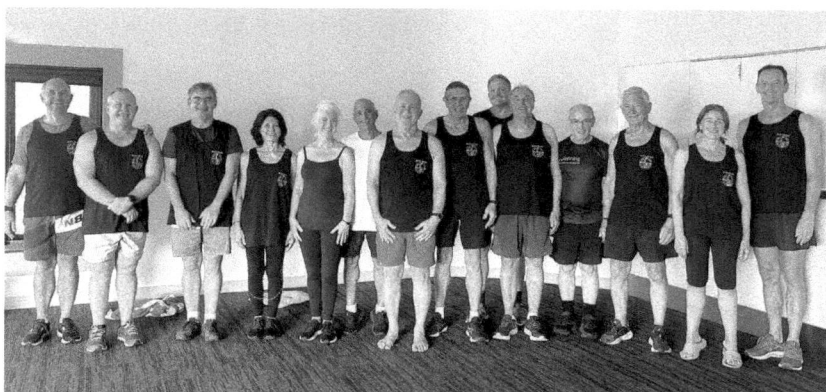

The Ab Lab at North Bondi Surf Club

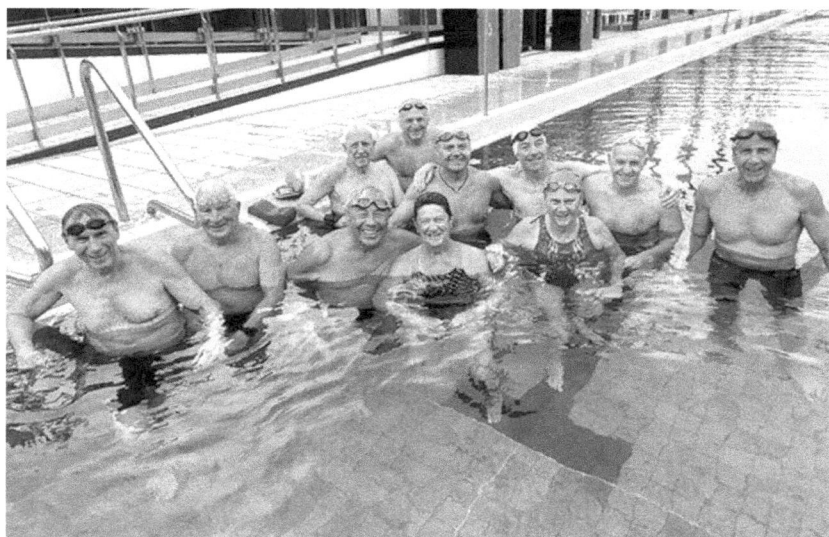

A Swim Squad at Moore Park

While the above tables are oriented towards the gym and weights, as we are seeking to retain muscle mass, the format can be similar for running, swimming and surf ski paddling. If it's running, it may be walk for five or 10 minutes, jog or run for 30 or 40 minutes followed by a jog and walk for five or 10 minutes. With swimming, it might be a warm-up 300m swim and kicking, 2 x sets of 600m (3 x 200m and/or 6 x 100m) and a warm down session up to 2km. Ski paddling and rowing can follow a similar pattern, generally keeping the time frame of about an hour.

Aerobics, yoga, Pilates

Aerobics, spin classes, yoga and Pilates can all form part of your PEP. The goal at the end of the day is to maintain muscle mass, bone density and keep all of the limbs and joints working. If we can achieve these three critical goals then it is likely we will have good strength, flexibility, balance and VO2. It is worth noting that bone density is built and maintained by high impact, weight-bearing exercise. It is worth trying all of these, to see which ones you like.

HIIT

I was previously of the opinion that there were injury and health risks for older people pursuing the HIIT type of training. However, my opinion has changed in the past five years, and I have been including HIIT in my training sessions with some identifiable benefits. A study in the *Journal of Physiology* in 2017 analysed the benefits of various forms of exercise for older adults, the HIIT method was found to be particularly effective.[75] Using an accepted HIIT training protocol developed

---

75 Wyckelsma, V.L., Levinger, I., McKenna, M.J., Formosa, L.E., Ryan, M.T., Petersen, A.C., Anderson, M.J., & Murphy, R.M. (2017). Preservation of skeletal muscle mitochondrial content in older adults: relationship between mitochondria, fibre type and high-intensity exercise training. *The Journal of Physiology*, 595(11), 3345–3359. https://doi.org/10.1113/JP273950 (Wyckelsma et al., 2017).

by Wisløff and colleagues, the exercise includes a three-minute warmup, one-minute active rest on a cycle ergometer; then four bouts of four-minute exercise intervals performed at an intensity corresponding to 90-95% of the heart rate peak.[76] Each interval was interspersed by four minutes of active recovery where participants cycled at 50-60% peak heart rate. The training session was concluded with a five-minute cool down. The HIIT training exercise was found to be highly effective in the preservation of mitochondrial content in skeletal muscles in older adults.[77] I now try and include at least one HIIT session a week. A starting HIIT option might be 4x1-minute effort with one-minute active rest between, and building up to the 4x4-minute protocol.

In December 2023, I turned 78. The ABS confirms that most people 75 and over are sedentary and on multiple forms of medication. To celebrate my 78th birthday, I swam 78x50m laps in a pool, with a few friends, in 78 minutes. This was a personal best for me at that age. My long-term goal for the following year was to compete in the Australian Surf Life Saving Masters Championships at Maroochydore, which I did, and I will discuss it in Chapter 8.

At the start of my 80th year, in the spirit of Jack LaLanne, I set myself two short- and two medium-term goals. My two

---

76 Wisløff, U., Støylen, A., Loennechen, J.P., Bruvold, M., Rognmo, Ø., Haram, P.M., Tjønna, A.E., Helgerud, J., Slørdahl, S.A., Lee, S.J., Videm, V., Bye, A., Smith, G.L., Najjar, S.M., Ellingsen, Ø., & Skjaerpe, T. (2007). Superior cardiovascular effect of aerobic interval training versus moderate continuous training in heart failure patients: A randomized study. *Circulation*, 115(24), 3086–3094.
77 Wyckelsma et al., 2017.

short-term goals were strength-related – lifting more than my body weight in a deadlift and twice my weight in a leg press. As mentioned, most 80-year-olds have lost more than 40% of their strength and muscle mass. I have never lifted anywhere near these weights before and, in fact, never done deadlifts. My weight at that time was 77kg. After a three-month build up, I managed three deadlifts (80kg) and five leg presses (160kg). These two short-term goals set me up for my medium-term goals, which were skiing powder for seven days in Japan and successfully competing in the Aussie Championships in the 1km soft sand run. Finally, I am part of an ageing study at UNSW (CHeBA, MAS 2). Part of the study was to measure grip strength, which is one of the tests for ageing. My measurements were 48kg for the left hand and 46kg for the right hand, which I was told was a good reading for a fit 40-year-old. As Jack LaLanne and Professor Maria Fiatarone Singh have shown, I wanted to prove you can maintain or improve your strength at 80, and that age is not a barrier to physical achievement. Similarly, like Jane Fonda, I feel younger and healthier now than I did in my 20s. Achieving these goals, at my age or any age, was only possible by preparing and sticking with my PEP. My remaining long-term goals for this year are completing this book, making my website more interactive, and doing more skiing.

A lifetime regime of exercise results in what has been described as 'biological capital', which is a benefit going forward that will support you through times of unwellness or injury. Human biological capital refers to an individual's accumulated biological resources, experiences and adaptations that influence their health, wellbeing and life changes. It encompasses inherited traits, epigenetic changes and the effects of early life and life-course experiences on biological systems.[78]

Your biological capital – built up over a lifetime of healthy living, regular vigorous exercise, good diet and nutrition, and consistent sleep – can help to lower blood pressure and cholesterol levels and ultimately a lower biological age. Socrates believed the body to be the foundation upon which a person builds their life and potential. In essence, he saw physical strength as an integral part of a well-rounded and fulfilling life, urging individuals to strive to reach their full potential in all aspects of their being. In my opinion, you can start collecting this biological capital at any age, with a consistent and programmed approach to exercise and healthy eating.

Review, refresh and reprogram

It is important to have a recovery week after a four-week solid PEP. During this week, you don't stop exercising, but you do back everything off – some weights, more stretching and abs, and have a day where you do nothing. You might also change the emphasis of your training, move to more legs or more swimming or play some more golf.

Remember your PEP is guided by your goals and what you hope to achieve in the short-, medium- and long-term.

---

78 Vineis, P. & Kelly-Irving, M. (2019). Biography and biological capital. *European Journal of Epidemiology*, 34, 979–982. https://doi.org/10.1007/s10654-019-00539-w

In summary, I argue that even a low level of exercise will help to improve the way you function and move about throughout the day. A person with a low level of activity will be better off than someone who is sedentary; however, they will still be prone to the various risk factors and have the potential for some form of disease. A slightly higher level of exercise will produce a greater amount of functionality, an increased level of cell rejuvenation and provide some protection against the various risk factors. It is also likely that there would be a lesser risk of disease with a subsequent reduction in risk factors.

A high level of exercise on a daily basis encourages the repair and regeneration of the cells within our body that keeps our cells on the growth path. This final level is a commitment to something like the PEP approach, with our short-, medium- and long-term goals firmly fixed in our exercise program. Rather than the inevitable decay, the cells are continually regenerating and replacing each other. In growth mode, we minimise both behavioural and biological risk factors and greatly reduce the risk of death from disease and cancer. Exercise may not be the fountain of youth, however it is the closest thing to a panacea for remaining as young as you can, for as long as you can.

In the next chapter we will look at the critical importance of sleep for our health, habits for optimal sleep, get to know more about our backs and how to prevent back pain, appreciate that rehab can be successful at any age ... and I discuss my last 'rodeo'.

Before you read on, pause and consider these two questions:

1. Would you like to be stronger at 80 than you were at 60 and lower your biological age?
2. Are you prepared to establish short-, medium- and long-term goals, then prepare and embark on a PEP?

CHAPTER 8: REHABBING THE BODY

As we have observed, the human body is like a machine that requires regular movement to function efficiently. It also requires fuel to provide energy, and rest and recuperation to allow our brains, cells, muscles and various parts to recharge. Most of us, who are active, would rather wear out than rust out.

On a daily basis we need regular sleep. It is critical that both these nightly and longer-term periods of rehabilitation of the body are faithfully pursued. Also, our spine has an important role to play in our wellbeing, yet most of us don't treat it with respect, until it demands attention. Finally, a bigger rehab commitment is required when we sustain a trauma or injury. The journey back after trauma is often daunting and can be prohibitive for many older people. Accordingly, this chapter will deal with sleep, the cleanser and rejuvenator, the important role your spine plays in your life, and the process of rehabbing and rebuilding muscle after injury.

Sleep – our brain's sewage system and body rejuvenator

Sleep is the sewage system for our brains and the rejuvenator of our body. Many biological processes occur during sleep. The brain stores new information and disposes of toxic waste. Nerve cells communicate and re-organise, which supports brain function. The body repairs cells, restores energy, and releases molecules like hormones and proteins. Sleep allows cells and muscles to repair and regrow. Parallel to this, the more you tear down the cells and muscles, the stronger they regrow, which in turn pushes back the biological clock.

My interviews with the Elders about their sleep habits were particularly revealing. All of the Elders were getting between seven and nine hours of quality sleep each night. They thought it was simply a given that a good night's sleep was essential for ageing successfully. They went to bed at a similar time each night, slept in a dark room and slept soundly. Also, they were all pursuing exercise regularly, if not daily. They were also pursuing many of the recommended sleep protocols without knowing it.[79]

In contrast, as your quintessential teenager, I had no idea about good sleep habits and thought that sleep was dispensable, or something I could catch up on when there was a lull in activities. In these younger days, I would have a late night, and play football or compete in a surf carnival the following day. I can recall on one occasion staying up all night and going straight to a footy game the following day. Surprisingly, I had a particularly good game.

At that age, I thought I was 10 feet tall and bulletproof. My appreciation for sleep improved slightly when I started university. I would get up at 3am, study for two hours, do a milk run with an incredibly fit mate, who we called the Machine, go for a surf, and then go to my day job. Like many younger people, I

---

79 Centre for Clinical Interventions. *Sleep hygiene.* https://cci.health. wa.gov.au

thought, 'there is plenty of time for sleep when you are dead'. I didn't realise that death comes much sooner to those with bad sleep habits. It wasn't until my late 20s and early 30s – when I was training and competing seriously – that I appreciated the importance of sleep.

In my senior years, at the tender age of 80, I am continually reminded how well I feel after a good night's sleep, compared to when I have a shocker! After a bad night's sleep, I am less organised, less coherent and less efficient in my daily activities. It's only when you look at the purpose of sleep and its importance in your blueprint for successful ageing that you prioritise it in your daily curriculum.

I have reviewed some of the information provided by experts in the field of sleep and now present some of the key reasons why good sleep is so important to successful ageing.

Firstly, let's consider the metabolic process. Sleep is closely linked to hormonal and metabolic regulation, allowing the body to conserve energy when it is least efficient to find food. In essence, sleep acts as the body's natural energy regulator – slowing metabolism when resources are scarce and restoring balance so we can function efficiently when awake.

While we sleep, the body undertakes vital cellular repair. Growth hormone is released, restoring tissues and regenerating muscle. Sleep also benefits brain function by consolidating memory, enhancing cognitive performance, clearing waste products, and supporting emotional balance and appetite control.

The relationship between sleep and diabetes is complex. Many people with type 2 diabetes experience poor sleep quality, making adequate rest essential for managing the condition. Sufficient sleep supports insulin function and blood sugar regulation, while sleep deprivation increases insulin resistance and raises blood glucose levels.

Sleep is also critical for immune and cardiovascular health. It strengthens immune cell activity, supports immunological memory, regulates cytokine production, and enhances the body's adaptive response. At the same time, it allows the heart and vascular system to rest and recover from the demands of the day.

Finally, as a competitor for many years, I can personally attest that consistent quality sleep can lead to greater athletic performance (while consistent bad sleep certainly won't do it any favours). Sleep significantly impacts on athletic performance, offering benefits in areas like speed, strength, endurance, accuracy and reaction time. Adequate sleep enhances muscle recovery and energy restoration, crucial for power and strength. Furthermore, it improves cognitive functions like focus, decision-making and sensory perception, leading to better neuromuscular coordination and faster responses.

My recent interview with Noah Havard, K4 Olympic silver medallist in Paris, found that these athletes were getting eight hours sleep each night and they were often having a nap in the afternoon.

I do not propose to discuss the four stages of sleep that we drift in and out of each evening; however, it does make for interesting reading.

The art of sleeping

I would like to discuss a few techniques for improving sleep as we age. We all have occasions when we have difficulties sleeping: it may be work problems, financial issues or emotional stress that we relive when we go to bed. I recall numerous times during my professional career 'sweating the small stuff' at night. Minor problems can become major ones, molehills become mountains, and campfires become bushfires when we put our head on the pillow. Numerous studies have identified processes that can improve the quality of your sleep. Recalling our discussion about habits in the previous chapter, my sleep habits are discussed below.

Sleep habits

My sleep habits have changed considerably over the last 80 years. As I mentioned, as a 20-year-old I didn't consider sleep to be important; and when I started studying, I would fit sleep into my schedule. On reflection, getting up at 3am to study, then doing a milk run, going for a paddle and going to work was very demanding and sleep was a low priority.

Now that I am not working a real job, my sleep pattern is far more regularised. I go to bed and get up early and normally sleep well. While my sleep habits may not be suited to others, they do seem to follow the established guidelines for good sleep hygiene.

The Sleep Health Foundation makes the following recommendations when it comes to sleep hygiene:

- Keep regular bedtimes and wake-up times – even on weekends – to help stabilise the body's internal clock and support better sleep.
- Limit screen use (TV, smartphones, tablets) one to two hours before bed and engage in relaxing, low-stimulus routines to wind down.
- Create a sleep-friendly environment: cool, dark, quiet, and reserved only for sleep (not work or entertainment).[80]

My sleep habits are as follows.

Pre-sleep routine

My pre-sleep routine starts about two hours before bed and includes not drinking coffee and alcohol and not eating food. This gives my digestive system a chance to work, and my stomach won't feel overloaded when I go to bed. Half an hour before I retire, I do some stretching, use a roller on the floor and generally relax. While I am using the roller, I also slow my breathing down and breathe in through the nose and out through the mouth.

Sleep environment

My wife and I have created a sleep environment that suits our needs. We like a dark room, with a cool temperature (21-22°C), with our watches and phones on silent. I also use eye

---

80 Sleep Health Foundation. *Sleep hygiene: Good sleep habits*. https://www.sleephealthfoundation.org.au/sleep-topics/sleep-hygiene-good-sleep-habits/

shades to make the room black. We both have a preferred pillow arrangement.

Sleep pattern

My sleep pattern is regular to the extent of being boring. I start heading to bed at about 8.45pm and try to be in bed by 9-9.15pm. My body clock normally wakes me between 4.30am and 5am and I seldom need the alarm. This can be frustrating on occasions when I am tired and I have decided that I would like to sleep in, to say, 6am.

Vitamins

I normally take my vitamins in the morning. However, if I've had a big day exercising, I may have a magnesium tablet going to bed as it helps to relax tired muscles and also helps me to sleep well.

Naps

I admit to succumbing to the temptation of a 30-minute nap, sometimes, in the afternoon, particularly if I have had two training sessions. However, I try and ensure it is early in the afternoon, so it doesn't interfere with my evening sleep.

Sleep position

As a result of injuries and surgery I have experimented with a number of sleep positions. After surgery on sequential shoulders, I was forced to sleep on my back. My wife complained that my snoring was excessive and that I was stopping breathing through the night. I was pleased to find this problem stopped as soon as I could start sleeping on my side. Firstly, sleeping on my right side after my left shoulder surgery; and secondly, sleeping on my left side after my right shoulder surgery.

In summary, a recent research study of over 173,000 adults concluded that men who got adequate sleep lived five years longer, while women who got adequate sleep lived two years longer. I really was incredibly naïve when I was young, and fortunate that treating sleep with such a lack of respect has not had any major health problems for me.[81]

Preventing back pain

Chronic back pain is one of the most debilitating health problems a person can encounter and as many as 80% of us will experience some form of back pain over a lifetime. Approximately four million (16%) of people in Australia were living with back problems in 2022. Of those, 72% were living with one or more other chronic conditions, with the most common comorbidities being mental and behavioural conditions (43%), arthritis (34%),

81 Rawlinson, K. (2023, February 23). Good quality sleep can add years to people's lives, study suggests. *The Guardian*. https://www.theguardian.com/society/2023/feb/23/good-quality-sleep-can-add-years-to-peoples-lives-study-suggests

and asthma (17%).[82] Back pain was worse among people in lower socio-economic areas, and in regional areas. Back problem expenditure in the health system accounted for $3.4 billion in 2020-21.

While a proportion of back pain results from a trauma, the majority is a result of lifestyle, including too much time on the couch or bent over a computer screen.

The spine is the major structural element that allows the back to function. It comprises five sub-structural elements, including the cervical spine, thoracic spine, the lumber spine, the sacrum and the coccyx, and these are shown in Figure 8.1.

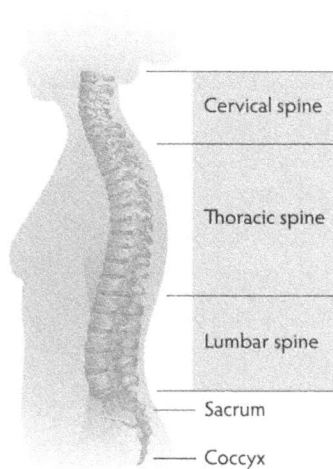

Cervical spine

Thoracic spine

Lumbar spine

Sacrum

Coccyx

Figure 8.1: The Spine, Sacrum and Coccyx.
Source: Modified image from Wikimedia Commons

---

82 AIHW. (2024). *Back problems.* https://www.aihw.gov.au/reports/chronic-musculoskeletal-conditions/back-problems

Know a little about your back

As you can see from the above diagram, the back is an important piece of super-structure that allows us to stand vertically and perform multiple movements. Ligaments and tendons are fibrous bands of connective tissue that are attached to bone. Ligaments connect two or more bones together and stabilise joints. Tendons attach muscle to bone and allow us to move our limbs.

Ligaments

The system of ligaments in the vertebral column combines with the tendons and muscles to provide a natural brace, to help protect the spine from injury. Ligaments aid in joint stability during rest and movement and prevent injury from hyperextension and hyperflexion (excessive movements).

Sitting for long periods of time or not having a strong core causes problems with the spine that can result in back pain. If ligaments or tendons become stressed or damaged, the surrounding nerves respond, causing a chain reaction, with muscles going into spasm to protect the injured area.

I have recently purchased a stand-up desk, which has helped my posture and burns more calories. In my early 40s, I thought I had a strong core as I did numerous sit-ups. It was not uncommon for me to do 1000 sit-ups with a medicine ball, in a session. However, I was not strengthening the core per se, the tiny muscles that support our spine in the critical locations: I was only building a 'six-pack'. I was ski paddling four times a week, and after training, I would experience severe back pain that was totally debilitating. I would become nauseous with the pain and could not find a comfortable position where the pain would dissipate.

I would be at work, and halfway through a meeting, I would have to lay on the floor. I was on the treatment treadmill for over six months – going from physio to physio and back expert to back expert. It was only after reading and learning about these tiny core muscles that support the spine that I was able to develop an abdominal (ab) routine to strengthen those muscles and the pain subsided. Now, I religiously do my core-based abs (at least 300) every morning, before heading out. My recommendations to avoid back pain are:

- Do 10-15 minutes of back neutral exercises each morning.
- Stretch hamstrings at least every second day.
- Don't sit for longer than an hour anywhere without standing and stretching.
- When you have developed some core strength, you can do 2-minute planks and strengthen your obliques, with 30 second oblique planks, each side.
- Stretching should be part of daily activities.
- Get a stand-up desk if you work in an office environment. It is the best investment I've ever made.

You may tell me you have no time for more exercise. But if you have had serious back pain you will readily agree that this is a small investment for a lifetime free of back pain!

Rehab can be successful at any age

The body has an amazing ability to recover from all types of traumas and injuries. As a long-time competitor, one of my philosophies is, if you are not living life on the edge you are taking up too much space! However, when you live life on the edge you occasionally fall off. I have participated in numerous sports, torn countless muscles and had numerous injuries. Recently, I tore a calf muscle skiing and after 12 weeks of leg rest and rehab, I am now able to walk but not yet able to run.

I have discovered the benefits of a good physiotherapist, and the importance of properly rehabilitating injured parts of the body. My go-to guy is Albert Alonso at Bondi Physio. Although I have had many sporting injuries, I managed to avoid the surgeon's knife until I was 70, when I tore the supraspinatus tendon off the bone in my left shoulder, while trying to paddle through a two-metre wave on my surf ski in 2020. These tendons make it possible to lift your arm and are often referred to as the rotator cuff.

I thought that I knew something about rehab until I had this injury. When my sports doctor and good friend, Dr John Best, gave me his diagnosis, that my injury was a torn rotator cuff, I was shattered. It would be a whole new world after surgery, trying to build back atrophied muscles and tendons that had wasted away during the six weeks when my arm was in a sling, then six months healing.

To add insult to injury, my left shoulder surgery was to be the first in a series of surgeries that I would need in my early 70s. As

I have always said, life is all about timing! My first surgery was to attach the supraspinatus and bicep tendon in the left shoulder, two days before St Vincents Private Hospital, was to be closed down and quarantined for COVID-19. After the surgery, I had an adverse reaction to the anaesthetic resulting in an enlarged prostate and retention, when you cannot pass urine, a most unpleasant experience. As the hospital was about to be closed, I had one hour to make a choice of prostate surgery or heading home with urinal tubing, that I may need for several months, until the hospital reopened. I chose prostate surgery with a spinal injection, which meant I was semi-awake during the process, not one of my better decisions. On returning home I was out of it for a few days after surgery and anaesthetic on two consecutive days. I had purchased a stationary bike for rehab, while my shoulder was recovering, however after prostate surgery I could not sit on my bike for three months. After 14 months of rehab and training, when I jumped on the double ski at the Aussie Championships in April 2021 for a warm-up and tore the same tendons in the right shoulder, it was truly demoralising. It was like *Groundhog Day*, I tore exactly the same tendons in the right shoulder; I would have the same surgery, same surgeon – except to a different shoulder. This time I did not have retention, however after the surgery, I had a chronically stiff neck and could not turn my head. This resulted in two lots of rehab, one for the right shoulder and the other for the neck. Both were very slow to improve and are still a work-in-progress. Subsequently, I had surgery to remove a cataract, an ablation for atrial fibrillation (AF), and, hopefully, finally, surgery to rectify the recalcitrant macular in my right eye.

I was fortunate enough to have a great medical team, including my sports medicine doctor, a good surgeon, and a good physio, to guide my rehab, which I followed meticulously. As patience is not one of my strong suits, it was particularly difficult to hold back from doing too much rehab too quickly.

Each of these surgeries required a different form of rehabilitation, with the shoulders being the most challenging. How footballers have surgery and are back on the field in months is beyond me. When I tore the first lot of tendons in the left shoulder, it was devastating as I was training for what I thought would be my last race. On reflection, it was funny when telling my surgeon how I tore my tendons. He replied, 'that is a great story, most people your age with this injury do it falling out of bed'. I took his comment as a perverse compliment. Also, on reflection, I recall listening to a group of older people, probably not as old as I am, talking about their operations and thinking, 'I hope I never get like that'. Well, I have!

However, I did learn the hard way that even a 70+ year-old person can build back muscle mass and strength, if they pursue a carefully prepared PEP and slowly increase resistance to the injured parts in the body. It is pointless trying to articulate a rehab program in this section as it depends on which part of the body you have injured. I can say it is not just a physical but also an emotional journey that you travel through with any rehab. As my rehab ordeal was peculiar, I have written about it in detail below. It is a classic example of setting short-, medium- and long-term goals to meet a long-term outcome, then resetting them when things don't go to plan.

My last rodeo

I decided that I would have one last crack at competing in the surf ski events at the Australian Surf Life Saving Masters Championships, which were held at Maroochydore in April 2024. An ambitious, some say stupid, goal for a 78-year-old, who by then had had two lots of shoulder surgery and an ablation for AF. The last time I competed was at the Aussie Masters at Broadbeach in 2021, when I jumped on the double ski with my long-time doubles partner John for a warm-up, and tore the supraspinatus tendon off the bone, this time in the right shoulder. This was not the way I wanted to finish 60 years of competing on the single and double ski.

As I had a similar injury and surgery on the left shoulder in 2020, I was painfully aware of what was involved in the rehab process. Indeed, I had a vivid recollection of the frustrating process, starting with six weeks with the arm in a sling after surgery, and the endless strengthening of the arm and shoulder. I say endless, as I still do these exercises daily. During the first two months the shoulder atrophied to a frightening extent and building back muscle mass and strength at my age is a slow process requiring complete commitment. While I have few attributes, I am committed when I decide to pursue a goal, and with the guidance of my sports medicine guru and my then physio we commenced rehabilitation for a second time.

To paint the complete picture, I decided to have an ablation after my first shoulder surgery. Previously, while training in the pool with a couple of swimmers half my age, I pushed too hard, and my heart went totally out of sync. It was a frightening experience and at the time I thought I was having a heart attack. However, after consulting my then GP and cardiologist, I was informed that it was AF. After 12 hours in hospital my heart reverted to its normal pace without me having to go through the heart shocking reversion process. I had persevered with Tambocor and Cardizem for over 12 months; however, I hated taking any form of medication and the AF attacks were becoming more prevalent. If you've not had AF, you will not appreciate how scary and debilitating it can be, when your heart jumps from 50 to 150bpm and back in seconds. It also comes in various forms from very mild to very extreme. Mine was probably mid-strength.

After going out of sync one too many times, I decided to have an ablation. An ablation is closed heart surgery where wires are inserted inside and outside the heart through the groin and the so-called electrodes of the heart that cause AF are frozen. I can report that Dr Murray did an excellent job, and I have not had a recurrence, please God it stays that way. However, when you push yourself at training, AF is always lurking in the back of your mind.

During my 12 months of rehabilitation, my right shoulder responded agonisingly slowly, although my surgeon had warned me this shoulder would be a more frustrating process. As a further complication after the surgery, I had a chronically stiff neck. I could not turn my head to the right and swimming was out of the question. To solve this problem, I started swimming with a snorkel and built up to 2km in a session, three times a week. My neck was now a bigger problem than my shoulder and I was pursuing neck exercises daily. I also had a cortisone injection in the neck, which is not a pleasant experience, and did not deliver a great deal of relief.

Everyone including myself was full of fear and trepidation that my shoulders would not cope with the serious paddling program required to compete in the single and double ski in the Aussie Masters surf titles in 2024. Most thought I was just crazy. Both shoulders had been the subject of surgery to reattach the torn tendons, and I had enthusiastically pursued two 12-month rounds of rehabilitation.

While carrying out my second round of shoulder rehab, I had commenced soft sand running and my knees and joints seemed to be coping reasonably well. I thought that this could be a fallback if my shoulders weren't up to the rigors of ski training. However, I had strained my left hamstring, before running in the 1km NSW Masters titles in March 2024, which required a separate round of rehab and hamstring strengthening exercises. This was a further mental stress. Effectively this meant that I had three separate training programs: one for the soft sand, one for ski paddling and a rehab program for my hamstring.

To complete my total program, I was training twice most days, each session taking at least one hour (plus warm-up and cool down) and 30 minutes of rehab. I was paddling four days, running three days, weights two or three days, and swimming two days. I was also still conducting my Pilates and Ab Lab session on Monday mornings and doing my stretching and abs every morning. A program eminently doable for a 30- or

40-year-old; a bit more of a challenge for someone 78. Again, Jack LaLanne was my inspiration. A special thanks to my wife Vicki for putting up with me during this time.

On Race Day One, at the Aussie Masters titles in Maroochydore, my nerves were palpable. I hadn't slept that night and all I could think of was the pain I experienced at my last Aussie Championships three years earlier, when I jumped on the double ski and tore my supraspinatus tendon. The surf was challenging as I paddled out for my warm-up, and I had a distinct lack of confidence. Suddenly, a wave stood up on the shallow bank in front of me and swatted me like a fly and I was knocked off my ski. While this was annoying at the time, it was the best thing that could've happened as it snapped me out of my malaise and got me focusing on the moment! The single ski race is about 500m, starting from the beach, then around a triangle of three buoys, and back to the beach. I began my race well and I was with the leading group off the beach when we were hit by a series of waves. Another paddler and I managed to sneak over a particularly large wave. A number of the other paddlers were hit, with some losing their skis.

I was now in second place all the way back to the beach. Just before the finish line, a small wave I had caught spun my ski around and I was facing in the wrong direction. I then made the fatal mistake of trying to turn around instead of just paddling backwards over the finish line, and a number of paddlers passed me. I felt that I deserved second place, and I was bitterly disappointed, and again had a sleepless night.

Race Day Two began with the 1km soft sand run at

Mooloolaba. The 1km race is an out and back course consisting of 4x250m laps, along the beach, up from the water on the soft sand. Rique Miroshnik, my amazing coach, insisted that I do a 500m warm-up. I was reluctant as my hamstring was again giving me problems leading up to the event. Anyway, I did what I was told and felt absolutely terrible. On reflection, it is better to feel terrible in the warm-up rather than in the race. As the officials had included three other age groups in the race, I did not know who I was racing in the 75 years and over category.

When the gun went off, I got a good start and there were four or five in front of me at the halfway mark. At the 750m, I was passed by two runners, and I was not certain which age group they were. As I felt particularly strong and thought I could not risk them being in the same age group, I stretched out and managed to pass them and was subsequently declared the winner of my age group. I then had to rush off to race in the double ski, which was being held 4km up the road at Maroochydore.

The double ski race was a memorable experience in what was a more challenging surf than the previous day. Fortuitously, we decided to have a quick warm-up; again, thoughts of my rotator cuff trauma three years earlier at Broadbeach flashed through my mind. However, those thoughts were short-lived paddling out, when we realised we couldn't steer our ski, and we hit another double ski on a wave, with a second ski narrowly missing us. We returned to the beach and adjusted the steering, ready for the race. It was so fortunate we had decided to have a warm-up.

The double ski race is similar to the single ski course, except a little longer. When the gun went, we got a good start and by halfway out we were leading by three ski lengths. When a large wave stood up and broke on top of us, John was caught underwater and under the ski. My first thought was to pull him out and to the surface, which I did. He was okay, a little shaken and he had swallowed lots of water. We then turned the ski over, jumped on, and started paddling. While most of the double crews had also been wiped out, one crew, who were three lengths behind us, had bounced over the wave and were now five lengths in front of us.

As we turned the last buoy a large swell was building behind us. Before I could think about anything, John had lifted the rating and we were chasing down this swell, which turned into a 3m wave, breaking in one metre of water. As we came down the face of the wave, we were both laying back on the deck of the ski to prevent the nose from diving, which would've been the end of our race. After a few very anxious moments, the nose of the ski popped up and we were flying towards the beach and catching the leading crew. We nearly lost it a few times in the foam on the way back to the beach but managed to correct and stay straight, holding the wave all the way to the finish line, with a commentator calling us first. As it turned out we were given second by half a metre. Although first place would've been nice, we had a memorable last race after 60 years of competition. We both agreed that this was a great way to finish our last rodeo!

Since my last rodeo, I have competed at the NSW and Australian Championships in 2025, only in the 1km soft sand run, which I was fortunate enough to win. John had decided not to paddle, so I concentrated on the run. As my hamstring is still troublesome, I do not know whether I will compete again in 2026, as it gets harder each year. Also, I am now pursuing rehab for a severely torn calf I did snow skiing. Hopefully, I will be able to start back doing some easy runs soon. As 75 is the oldest age group there are 'young guys' coming up each year. It is difficult to give away five years at my age.

As we age, we regularly have parts that wear out or become injured. It is important to respond to these setbacks positively and some form of rehab may be required. Rehab is inevitable if you are training hard; at some stage you will need it. If you have an injury or a health setback, don't respond by giving up your goals. Work through the problem, pursue the rehab, adjust your short- and medium-term goals and refocus on your long-term goals!

• • •

In summary, the human body is continually in rehab mode, whether it is cleansing and rejuvenating during sleep or in a more involved form of rehab responding to injury. However, we can do much to prevent injuries from occurring by sleeping regularly and looking after our spines, muscle system, tendons, organs and other parts. Australians who enjoy sitting on the lounge are most vulnerable in the spinal region and I caution everyone to treat their back with the respect that it deserves. We need to look after our bodies; it is the only place we have to live.

In the next chapter we will look at addictions, risk factors that might prevent healthy, successful ageing, and examine whether our uptake of unhealthy habits such as drinking, gambling, smoking or consuming fast foods might be influenced by vested interests.

Before you read on, pause and consider these two questions:

1. Are you getting seven hours or more of good sleep each night? Are you prepared to pursue some of the techniques mentioned previously to improve your sleep?

2. Are you experiencing back problems? Have you tried any of the previously mentioned back exercises? If not, are you prepared to give them a go?

CHAPTER 9: ADDICTIONS, RISK FACTORS AND VESTED INTERESTS

This chapter has three separate related components that collectively influence our approach to ageing. The first section considers addictions that destroy people's lives, and I raise the question of whether there are such things as healthy addictions. The second section revisits risk factors with a slightly different perspective, and considers how our own behaviour can determine how we age and potentially whether we will have heart disease or suffer from cancer. The final section deals with my theory on vested interests, which I foreshadowed in the introduction, and the way these culprits covertly work together to keep us unhealthy.

Addictions

There are many addictions recognised by health experts that have major impacts on mental and physical health, which in turn can affect our daily lives. Health professionals readily identify tobacco, drugs, alcohol and gambling as creating major problems. Health professionals are less enthusiastic to identify sugar, fast foods and mobile phones, which I have included. Also, controversially, I have identified prescription medication as an addiction for the medical profession, many older people and pharmaceutical companies. Let's discuss a few facts about these addictions and consider if any are actually good for us.

Tobacco

Tobacco has been the most insidious addiction, historically, as it was promoted as being 'cool and safe' for consumers, while the devastating effects from smoking were withheld by the cigarette companies. Evidence showing lung and other cancers that resulted from smoking was continually refuted by the tobacco lobby. The cigarette advertising was compelling for many. The 'Marlboro Man', and the 'Anyhow* have a Winfield' campaigns are just samples of the way cigarettes were promoted in the 70s and 80s.

When I was born in 1945, historic statistics showed that three out of four males and one in four females were smokers.[83] When I was a child, my father would smoke 40 cigarettes on a normal day. Although he gave up smoking 'cold turkey' at the age of 40 following a dire health warning from his doctor, when he passed away at 85, it was smoking that had done the damage. In contrast, my dear Mum smoked one or two cigarettes a day (she called them 'punkers', which I think was a Mumism for puffing), until she passed away at the age of 96. She did smoke a few more 'punkers' in her final year with the onset of dementia: she would complain about not having had a smoke for months, when she had just put one out.

A number of successful government-driven public awareness campaigns have brought about a dramatic reduction in smoking habits. The AIHW reports that among people aged 14 and over

---

83 Scollo, M.M., & Winstanley, M.H. (2012). *Tobacco in Australia: Facts and issues*. (4th ed). Cancer Council Victoria. www.TobaccoInAustralia. org.au

the proportion who smoked daily more than halved from 24% in 1991 to 8.3% in 2022-2023.[84] However, e-cigarettes and vaping are promoted as a soft alternative. According to the Australian Cancer Council, statistics indicate that young people who try e-cigarettes are three times more likely to take up smoking than those who have never vaped.[85]

Smoking is the worst health risk you can pursue, as it causes cancer, heart disease and many other problems. Nationwide health risks from smoking have been reduced with the reduction in the number of people smoking. The population has become increasingly aware of the general health impacts and likely risk of cancer for smokers. However, vaping and illicit tobacco is the next potential health risk.

Drugs

According to data from the most recent AIHW National Drug Strategy Household Survey 2022-23, around one in five (18% or 3.9 million) people over the age of 14 in Australia used an illicit drug in the previous 12 months. Concerningly, this is an increase from 2013, where 15% of people in Australia reported recent use of an illicit drug.[86] This includes cannabis, ecstasy, methamphetamine (street name ice), cocaine, hallucinogens, and

---

84 AIHW. (2025). *Alcohol, tobacco & other drugs in Australia*. https://www.aihw.gov.au/reports/alcohol/alcohol-tobacco-other-drugs-australia/contents/drug-types/tobacco

85 Cancer Council Australia. (2023). *E-cigarettes and vaping*. https://www.cancer.org.au/cancer-information/causes-and-prevention/smoking/e-cigarettes

86 AIHW. (2025). *National drug strategy household survey 2022-2023*. https://www.aihw.gov.au/reports/illicit-use-of-drugs/national-drug-strategy-household-survey/contents/summary

heroin. Although illegal, drugs in various forms are promoted to the vulnerable in our society, normally resulting in catastrophic effects. There are many reasons why someone may resort to taking drugs. These reasons might be personal or professional problems or simply peer pressure. In any case, my message is find other ways to get your high. Exercise, as I have set out in previous chapters, is an excellent alternative.

If you are encouraged to take any form of drugs, think about the long-term impact, rather than any perceived short-term benefit.

Gambling

As a total non-gambler, with the exception of the Melbourne Cup sweeps, I've never seen the sense in it, as you can never win. However, approximately 46% of the Australian population disagree with me (according to the AIHW's 2023 *Gambling in Australia* report), and gambling is identified as a risky behaviour. The forms of gambling identified include lotteries/scratches (64%), horse-racing (38%), sports betting (34%), and pokies (33%). Approximately 70% of the roughly one in two Australians who gamble do it across multiple forms. The real problem with gambling is that the government and gambling organisations are the main ones making money from these activities.

Gambling is one of the fastest growing addictions, and it has never been so widely advertised as it is currently. We are encouraged to bet with loved ones, friends and syndicates, not just on the outcome of a game or race, but on multiple facets of any given activity, which can potentially result in the player

MY BLUEPRINT FOR SUCCESSFUL AGEING

losing considerable money. Australians lost $25 billion on legal forms of gambling in 2019, representing the largest per capita losses in the world.[87]

While this is not meant to be a sermon, gambling is one of the most useless and potentially dangerous past times you can pursue.

Fast food

Fast food is one of the great addictions that has changed society with the corruption of the Australian diet by the US fast food companies. Many different books and documentaries have tracked the growth in overweight and obesity worldwide, following the spread of Coca-Cola, McDonald's, and other fast food multinationals. In a four-week period, in Australia, McDonald's had 8.1 million customers, KFC 6.8 million, Hungry Jack's 4.2 million, and Domino Pizzas 4.1 million. The lesser lights were Subway (3.2 million) and Red Rooster (2.1 million). As part of this study, those customers attended at least once.[88]

In my view, fast food contributes to Australia being one of the fattest countries in the world. On a recent drive, I stopped at one of these outlets to use the bathroom and was taken aback by the grotesque images of hamburgers and food displayed above the counter. I felt like I was putting on weight, just looking at

---

87 AIHW. (2023). *Gambling in Australia*. https://www.aihw.gov.au/reports/australias-welfare/gambling

88 Roy Morgan Research. (2021, May 24). *McDonald's, KFC, Hungry Jack's & Domino's Pizza are Australia's favorite restaurants*. https://www.roymorgan.com/findings/mcdonalds-kfc-hungry-jacks-dominos-pizza-are-australias-favorite-restaurants

196

these signs. While this problem is endemic in Australia, it has become worse with the introduction of delivery services that will deliver any form of fast food you want, almost at any hour of the day or night. It is a shame to see young people getting Macca's delivered for breakfast. It is sad for two reasons: firstly, they won't get off their ass and walk to the shop, and secondly that they chose to have that type of brekkie. The ominous truth is that the number of overweight or obese people is on the increase!

Mobile phones and social media

Mobile phones and social media can be addictive – just look at how many people are on their phones the next time you are at a bus stop – with some overlap between problematic smartphone use and problematic social media use. Australia's appetite for mobile phones follows the pattern of growing worldwide demand. About 88% of Australians own a mobile phone according to a 2021 study.[89] A 2022 Deloitte survey found more than nine out of every 10 Australians owns a smartphone.

Social media has connected everyone and made us friends with no one. On a sunny day at Bondi there are thousands of people on the promenade and almost all of them are on their mobile phone. Very few of these people are enjoying the moment. Smartphones have become deeply embedded in everyday life. We use them for almost everything – from work and communication to entertainment, banking and social

---

89 Linden, T., Nawaz, S., & Mitchell, M. (2021). Adults' perspectives on smartphone usage and dependency in Australia. *Computers in Human Behavior Reports*, *3*, 100060. https://doi.org/10.1016/j.chbr.2021.100060

connection. For many people, checking the phone has become an automatic habit, filling the quiet moments between tasks. Social media, streaming and messaging platforms now occupy a large part of our attention, shaping how we spend time, connect with others and even rest.

Mobile phone technology has advanced to a point where these devices can do almost anything. However, these benefits come with a cost. Our population has become more sedentary and much fatter. We have increased heart-related diseases and an increase in the number of cancer cases. Have you ever considered having a fasting day, not from food, but from your phone? Your level of mobile phone usage determines your level of addiction. Is it healthy or unhealthy?

The growing addiction to mobile phones and social media has made numerous suppliers millionaires and many Aussies sedentary. One day a week away from your phone could be the starting point to improve your lifestyle.

Prescription medication

Prescription medication has become one of the most lucrative sources of income for pharmaceutical companies (Big Pharma). A reasonable person might ask – do we need all of the medications that are prescribed, and is it making us healthy or unhealthy? On moving my dear old Mum from the Central Coast to Bondi, my role as a carer intensified from part-time to full-time and my first task was to review her medication. Although I'm not a medical doctor, I have researched the impacts of long-term use of various forms of medication. Also, my interviews with health professionals and Elders provided some real-life case studies of the use of medication.

As I mentioned in the introduction, Mum was taking 12 different types of medication prescribed by at least three different doctors, which immediately raised my concern as to whether all of these drugs were necessary. Accordingly, I organised an appointment with a GP, who specialised in older people. The short story is the GP reduced the number of prescribed medications from 12 to four. The experience with my Mum revealed that additional prescribed medications were included in her regime without reviewing the whole package.

Statins are the most lucrative form of prescribed medication on the market. Since the introduction of statins by Pfizer in the 1980s, it has become one of the most profitable drugs in the history of medicine. With increased competition, the cumulative revenue from statins from those first early sales in the US reached $US1 trillion by 2020.

Statins are very big business. Most prescribed medications, particularly statins, become addictions, for patients and the pharmaceutical companies: patients because they are told they must stay on the drugs for a lifetime, and the pharmaceutical companies as they are making obscene profits. Clearly statins are life saving for some. The question is, are these drugs improving our health or undermining it? Are we healthier than we were in the 1980s or are we sicker?

There are many drugs with a similar storyline. We are probably guilty of creating this dilemma. When we go to the doctor, we expect them to give us a prescription, otherwise we feel we have not got our money's worth. The issue with our health system is the lack of focus on preventative medicine and the lack of training for the medical professionals on the benefits of exercise and a healthy diet. Wouldn't it be healthier if doctors were prescribing exercise with vegetables and fruit, in place of medicine, where possible? I will discuss some of my issues with modern medicine later in this chapter.

Alcohol

Alcohol is clearly a behavioural risk factor that needs to be identified. Statistics from the AIHW reveal 77% of Australians consume alcohol and one in two consume it at risky levels.[90] The estimated social cost of alcohol use in Australia was $66.8 billion in 2017-2018.[91]

Although governments have now required providers of alcohol to identify risks, governments are still making obscene money on excise and taxes from producers and suppliers of alcohol. Tax revenue and excise from alcohol was $7.5 billion in 2022-23, with many more millions lost due to underreporting and avoidance practices.[92] I admit to enjoying a cold beer, preferably Tooheys Old, and a glass or two of a good shiraz with dinner. Life is too short to not drink good wine. I do have at least one alcohol free day (AFD), each week, to prove I'm not alcohol dependent.

90 AIHW. *Alcohol*. https://www.aihw.gov.au/reports-data/behaviours-risk-factors/alcohol/overview
91 National Drug Research Institute. (2021, December 16). *The $67 billion cost of one of our favourite drugs*. Curtin University. https://ndri.curtin.edu.au/news-events/ndri-news/media-release-%2467-billion-cost-of-alcohol
92 ATO. (2024, November 1). *Latest estimate and trends: Alcohol tax gap*. https://www.ato.gov.au/about-ato/research-and-statistics/in-detail/tax-gap/a-h-tax-gaps/alcohol-tax-gap/latest-estimate-and-trends

I recall once being told by a lifestyle doctor that I was alcohol dependent. The doctor that was providing me with advice, who was recommended to me by a friend, was conservatively 10-15kg overweight. While I didn't say anything at the time, which surprised my wife, my thought was he should take some of his own advice. Although I am a hard marker, I think health professionals have less credibility when they don't practice what they preach. As this advice did cause me some concern, I did go and see my regular doctor and had a full set of blood tests, which were more than acceptable. You could question whether my indulgence is healthy or unhealthy. However, it does give me pleasure and at this stage it does not seem to be having any adverse impacts on my health. Recently, I had lunch with a friend who turned 95; he looked in good shape and is still as sharp as a tack. He enjoys a couple of Scotches each night. Our late Queen enjoyed a couple of gins each day and my old Mum enjoyed a 'tipple', with both passing at 96. I previously mentioned attending a friend's 100th birthday, where he enjoyed celebrating with wine.

There is no universally accepted 'safe' amount of alcohol consumption. While the Australian Guidelines recommend no more than 10 standard drinks per week and no more than four standard drinks on any one day, to reduce health risks, even within these limits, the risk of harm is still present. Risky levels of consumption of alcohol is clearly a problem. The question is whether a few drinks a day is harmful. There are strong and opposing views on this topic. I have often thought that a useful study might be comparing two similar individuals with similar diets doing similar levels of exercise. Individual A would consume three standard alcohol drinks a day, and Individual B would consume three sugary drinks a day, say 375ml cans, which would contain between 24-36 teaspoons of sugar in total. It would be interesting to see if either individual increased their waist and weight measurements or blood sugar levels after six months. I will also talk about sugary drinks later in this chapter.

Healthy addictions

Is there such a thing as a healthy addiction? Are all addictions bad for our health span, lifespan and family? Or are there some addictions that are pleasurable and provide us with a sense of reward or achievement?

An addiction is broadly defined as a compulsion to pursue an activity or consume a substance that brings about pleasure. If we take this somewhat generic definition, I have multiple addictions. First, I am addicted to water, more the ocean than the harbour or the river, and I must get my fix each day. I need to either swim in it, paddle on it or at least look at it! I find it restful, soothing, stress-relieving and stimulating. Indeed, it gives me great pleasure paddling my surf ski (another addiction) out through the break. It is liberating, euphoric and provides a feeling of escapism that is difficult to describe to someone who has not grown up at the beach and had the water as an intrinsic part of their life. Is this a healthy or unhealthy addiction?

My second addiction is exercise. However, it wasn't until I joined the surf club, my third addiction, that I realised that members down there ran, swam, paddled skis, and went to the gym to get fit as well as to save lives. It was in my formative days in the surf club where I became committed to exercising every day. It was then I started recording what I did in training and wanted to learn as much about exercise as I could. I went to courses, went to training clinics and completed coaching accreditation courses. I attended lectures on exercise, health and fitness and purchased every book available. I would write training programs for our ski paddling team and record the programs we pursued, and the results we obtained from competition. By any interpretation, this was clearly an addiction. It was firstly as a boat rower, then a beach sprinter, march past, ski paddler, and more recently a soft sand runner.

Does my addiction to exercise have risk factors? The clear answer is yes! I am notorious for overtraining. It's not that I purposely overtrain, it's simply that when I'm enjoying the moment, I keep thinking, 'well, I might just do one more set'. Someone asked me recently, 'Why do you do this?' The answer is simple, because I love it! Some say I'm addicted, my wife says I'm obsessive, and I like to think of it as just doing stuff I enjoy doing and which makes me feel good. My extended answer is, it's a lot healthier than drugs, gambling, smoking, sitting on the lounge or eating at McDonald's, and hopefully this addiction continues to keep me off medication.

Nutrition

Nutrition, otherwise referred to as diet, is my next positive addiction. I became interested in nutrition in my 30s and I got very close to pursuing a sports medicine degree; however, town planning was my professional passion, as I still thought I could change the world. Yet nutrition became a critical part of my life, and, like exercise, I could not get enough information about it. When I eventually got involved in my PhD, I experimented with all of the different diets that were touted as being healthy or unhealthy. My observations are noted previously in this book.

My adaptation of the Mediterranean diet is my choice, as it is rich in fibre, vegetables, healthy fats and anti-inflammatory foods. These can lower the risk of certain cancers. My version includes more oily fish, some grass-fed meat and no processed meat. The Mediterranean diet has been shown to improve mental health and quality of life. It can also reduce depression and cognitive decline. Nutrition is not rocket science! It is as simple as the 80:20 Rule – try and do the right thing 80% of the time and don't get too naughty during the other 20%. Items to avoid are: salt, sugar, dairy products and processed foods. Most of the time eat vegetables and lean protein and some fruit. It's as simple – and as difficult – as that! I have discussed my experience with nutrition and my diet previously in Chapter 6.

I have a cluster of addictions under the heading of food, and these are a natural extension of my obsession for nutrition. My four food addictions are homemade cereal, which I make myself, coffee, New Zealand salmon and lastly, I am mildly embarrassed to say, mashed potato.

I mentioned my cereal previously, so I won't discuss it further in this section except to say that it comprises fresh organic-grown produce, almost all of which is unrefined. The purpose of this brew is to clean and scour the bowel, feed the gut and replenish the body from exercise undertaken earlier that morning, while providing a concoction that I seriously enjoy. My cereal is splashed with soy milk and accompanied with a banana and yoghurt that share centre stage with the blackberries and blueberries, plenty of nuts and prunes.

Coffee is a great way to start the day! My wife can't make a move in the morning before she has her coffee. I try and wait until after I finish my first training session. It becomes my reward after a hard session. I can recall being in New York in 1988 when everyone was walking around with these large takeaway cups of coffee. I remember thinking to myself if you cornered the market for cups when this trend comes to Australia, you could make quite a lot of money. Sadly, that was another good idea that was not pursued. However, if I have coffee after lunchtime, it becomes a risk for my sleep pattern.

New Zealand Ora King salmon has had mixed publicity both good and bad. On the negative side, it has been reported the salmon are fed antibiotics and other supplements. However, I love the oily salmon and particularly if it is served rare. Vicki and I actually paddled a kayak around the largest salmon farms in New Zealand. These farms were massive in size, in very deep, free-flowing cold water and the salmon seemed very happy and healthy. My opinion is that there are many benefits from including red salmon, particularly Ora King, in your diet. Also, it does not seem to have the problems experienced by the Tasmanian salmon industry which have been reported in the media. Our preference is New Zealand Ora King salmon.

Finally, mashed potato takes a little bit more explaining as it is a passion. I grew up with mashed potato since my Mum started serving it to me, nearly 80 years ago. As mentioned, we were the traditional Aussie family, with a meat and three veg diet. Clearly, our current diet has changed, with a lot less meat, but the mashed potato has endured with some modifications, about three or four times a week. The butter and milk used to mash the potatoes has been replaced with soy milk, normally Bonsoy as it seems to have less sugar, and sometimes I add some olive oil. Could I live without it? Yes, I could, but I would miss it. Is it healthy or unhealthy? I'll leave that for others to decide. However, I do enjoy it, and I would like to think it forms part of my 80% tally!

Risk factors

It was once thought that the manner in which you aged was preordained by how carefully you selected your parents. It was thought that genetics would determine whether you aged successfully or suffered from early decrepitude. While research now confirms that genetics provides strong links to various diseases, it has only a 20-30% influence on the way in which we age. The remaining 70-80% is lifestyle.[93] While some of the complexities of healthy living have been discussed in other chapters, lifestyle has the most profound impact on the way we age.

In previous chapters we discussed how we measure ageing. There are two recognised methods for measuring how old we are. The first is chronological ageing, which is simply a record of

93 University of Oxford. (2025, February 20). *Lifestyle and environmental factors affect health and ageing more than our genes.* https://www.ox.ac.uk/news/2025-02-20-lifestyle-and-environmental-factors-affect-health-and-ageing-more-our-genes

how long you have been on this planet or how many birthdays you have celebrated. The second method is measuring biological age, which is the age of your body, your mind, and, indeed, your spirit. While you can't control your chronological age, you can influence your biological age.

William Evans and Irwin H. Rosenberg were prominent researchers in the field of ageing and nutrition science in the 1990s. Together, they co-authored the influential book *Biomarkers: The 10 Determinants of Ageing You Can Control*. Their book introduced the concept of 'biomarkers' – measurable indicators of physiological ageing – and emphasised the role of lifestyle interventions, particularly strength training, in promoting healthy ageing.

Their research at that time was groundbreaking, proving that biological ageing can be measured and slowed down by controlling body mass, strength, metabolic rate, body fat, aerobic capacity, sugar tolerance, cholesterol ratio, blood pressure, bone density, and the body's ability to regulate temperature. Subsequent research has shown that not only can the biological ageing process be slowed down, it can also be lowered (see 2004's *Younger Next Year: A Guide to Living Like 50 Until You're 80 and Beyond* by authors Chris Crowley and Henry S. Lodge, MD). Additionally, it is possible to add strength and vitality to your life at any age. At 80, I am lifting heavier weights now than ever before. The theory advanced in my work stands on the shoulders of these earlier researchers and similarly argues that controlling your biomarkers can control your biological ageing.[94]

---

94 See Bortz, 1991; Evans & Rosenberg, 1991; Paffenbarger & Olsen,

It follows that our biological ageing is directly related to our exposure to risk factors. These risk factors are many and varied, and if you are reading this book, I would make the broad assumption that you don't smoke or take illicit drugs. Behavioural risk factors can result in downstream biomedical risk factors, which impact on your biomarkers and can accelerate your biological ageing. High on this list of behavioural risk factors that we should avoid include physical inactivity and an unhealthy diet. If you are pursuing regular exercise and consuming healthy food, you have a much better chance of maintaining muscle mass, while controlling body fat, your waist measurement, and aerobic capacity. Controlling these markers can in turn help stabilise your sugar tolerance, cholesterol ratio, blood pressure, bone density and metabolic rate. If you can control your biomarkers as you move into your 60s, your biological age will be considerably less than your chronological age and you can greatly reduce your need for medication. Also, your strength is likely to be greater, and you will be less susceptible to the old person's curse – falling.

In Chapter 2, I identified what health professionals regard as the most frequently occurring risk factors both behavioural and biomedical. The top five in each category are as follows:

Behaviour risk factors

- lack of exercise, being sedentary – a disaster for mind and body, resulting in frailty;
- unhealthy diet, too little vegetables and fruit, too much refined/processed food;

1996; Robbins, 2006; Rowe & Kahn, 1998.

- sleep deficit, multiple downstream health impacts;
- drinking excessively (more than four standard drinks per day); and
- smoking, unwellness, cancer and heart disease.

Biomedical risk factors

- overweight and obesity;
- depression;
- diabetes;
- high cholesterol; and
- high blood pressure.

A final risk factor that I would briefly mention is stress, which can be in both camps. It can be a result of behaviour, an action we perpetrate, or it can be biomedical in response to circumstances beyond someone's control. It could be the loss of a loved one, a marriage break-up or financial loss that can be the trigger for depression, a heart attack, angina or other immune responses. Stress is often a camouflaged risk factor that we know little about and need to become more aware of.

In summary, it's important to understand the link between our behaviour and what happens in our bodies as we age. Perhaps if more people understand the potential repercussions of what they do, they may make more informed decisions.

In the following section we will explore why we are becoming increasingly unwell as we age. Are we the only ones to blame – or are there hidden factors at play?

A world of deception

I have a theory that we live in a world of deception that is driven by vested interest groups. Most of these interest groups (the culprits) that could help to improve our lifestyle as we age are driven by their own agenda. There are seven culprits in my theory, identified in the introduction, which I will now discuss further.

The food manufacturers are one of the leaders in this conspiracy. Their primary aim is to appeal to our palate, so we consume highly processed and unhealthy food and spend money. Their secondary aim is to hit the sweet spot in our ghrelin hormone (aka the 'hunger hormone') in our stomach with a combination of salt and sugar that tricks our brain into thinking we should eat more than we need. This problem is further compounded by the obscure information on the packaging.

How can it be said that a sugary drink containing 8-12 teaspoons (33-50g) of sugar or refined food with four to five additives or known carcinogens is healthy? The increased consumption of these products is enhanced by extensive advertising campaigns. According to the ABS National Health Survey 2020-21, 6.4% of adults consumed sugar sweetened drinks daily.[95] Meanwhile, the Australian Medical Association (AMA) says that 'Australians consume more than 2.2 billion litres of sugary drinks every year. That's enough to fill 880 Olympic sized swimming pools'. It also said in *Sickly Sweet*, its 2025-2026 Pre-Budget Submission, that 'in 2019-20, Australians

---

95 ABS. (2022). *Dietary behaviour.* https://www.abs.gov.au/statistics/health/food-and-nutrition/dietary-behaviour/2020-21

consumed on average 70 grams of free sugar a day, with more than a quarter (18g) of this coming from sugary drinks'.[96] This is only the tip of the iceberg and doesn't take account of the sugar added to most refined food.

Supermarkets are the next culprits in my theory. The sugary unhealthy drinks and products are in the central aisles and on the most accessible shelves. The healthy items are on the periphery on shelving that is less accessible. Clever marketing encourages us to purchase more of the sugary/salty products as they are discounted if we buy several packets. There are also end aisle items which command a premium for their location. These items, which are located at the end of an aisle in a prominent position or near the check-out, are invariably unhealthy and sugary, very attractive to children, and parents are cajoled into purchasing these items. My advice for visiting the supermarket is to shop the periphery and the vegetables and fruit section.

Modern medicine and the medical profession is the next on my list. Modern medicine has proved to be excellent in diagnosing and treating contagious diseases; however, it has been less successful responding to noncommunicable diseases (NCDs). The medical profession is trained to respond to symptoms like high blood pressure, high blood glucose and high blood lipid, but not the actual cause of any of these conditions.[97] For example, diets high in added sugar are referred to as Hyperinsulinemia and can result in leptin resistance, insulin resistance, and sodium

---

96 AMA. (2025) *Sickly sweet: What's the problem?* https://www.ama.com.au/sickly-sweet/whats-the-problem

97 Lustig, R. (2021). *Metabolical: The truth about processed food and how it poisons people and the planet.* Yellow Kite.

and fluid retention. Also, diets with between 10-24.9% of added sugars have a 30% higher risk of mortality from cardiovascular disease.[98] Importantly, high levels of added sugars and refined foods can adversely impact on metabolism and can lead to type 2 diabetes.

Metabolism is the set of life-sustaining chemical reactions that occur in living organisms. It involves converting food into energy to fuel all bodily functions, from breathing to thinking, and also includes building and repairing tissues. Essentially, it's the process by which your body turns what you eat and drink into the energy it needs to function. *Metabolical* author Dr Robert Lustig and others argue that when we consume large amounts of sugar and refined foods we are potentially moving towards a state of metabolic syndrome, which is a cluster of conditions that occur together, increasing the risk of chronic NCDs such as heart disease, stroke and type 2 diabetes.

A person is diagnosed with metabolic syndrome if they have at least three or more of the following risk factors – high blood pressure, high waist circumference, low levels of HDL 'good' cholesterol, high levels of blood triglycerides, insulin resistance or type 2 diabetes – according to the Victor Chang Cardiac Research Institute.[99] Type 2 diabetes and metabolic syndrome are associated with an increased risk of cancer. An estimated one

---

98 Yang, Q., Zhang, Z., Gregg, E.W., Flanders, W.D., Merritt, R., & Hu, F.B. (2014). *Added sugar intake and cardiovascular diseases mortality among US adults. JAMA Internal Medicine*, 174(4), 516–524. https://doi.org/10.1001/jamainternmed.2013.13563
99 Victor Chang Cardiac Research Institute. *Metabolic syndrome.* https://www.victorchang.edu.au/heart-disease/metabolic-syndrome

in 20 Australians live with undiagnosed diabetes. This figure includes those with type 1, type 2, and other forms of diabetes, but not gestational diabetes. Almost one in five Australians aged 80-84 (19%) live with diabetes – nearly 30 times the rate of those under 40 (0.7%). Between 2000 and 2021, the number of Australians living with diabetes rose almost 2.8-fold, from 460,000 to 1.3 million – a shocking figure, even taking into account population growth and an ageing population.[100] Using an analogy, should modern medicine be treating the downstream pollution or the upstream contaminators? Perhaps both, initially! However, if you can stop the upstream contaminators, you stop the downstream pollution.

Dr Lustig argues exercise, diet and lifestyle could resolve or prevent metabolic syndrome in most cases. However, most doctors are not trained in preventative medicine, and most doctors don't like telling their patients that they are overweight or obese and should do some exercise and lose weight. Instead, the practice is to prescribe Ozempic, which is the current weight loss craze. The side effects from this drug are just starting to be realised. My then GP, who I interviewed as part of my research, said to me, 'Doctors are not trained to keep you well, we are here to fix you up when you get crook'. He went on to add, 'when I did my degree, I had one lecture on food/nutrition and no lectures about exercise'. It is little wonder our health system is geared the way it is, with preventative medicine being the poor relation. As mentioned, it is a concern when the primary

---

100 AIHW. (2024). *Diabetes: Australian facts*. https://www.aihw.gov.au/reports/diabetes/diabetes/contents/summary

medical mission statement is 'to do no harm'! What if their mission statement was, to keep you well?

Big Pharma, a major player, wants us to take more drugs, whether we need them or not. Statins are one of the most profitable drugs on the market and everyone over the age of 50 is encouraged to take them to lower cholesterol. There are countless dollars spent on finding cures for various diseases, which I support. However, there are negligible amounts of money spent on finding the cause of these diseases so that we might avoid them in the first place. Would you prefer to be cured of cancer or to totally avoid it? The critical question our researchers should be pursuing is why there are more NCDs, neurological and heart diseases and numerous cancers than ever before. Is the increase in NCDs a function of our lifestyle or the poisons being added to processed food? Again, why is there such little financial support for preventative medicine? Is it the unfortunate truth that Big Pharma and the medical profession make more money when we are unwell?

The media also plays a critical role in this conspiracy. I recently watched an ABC-TV *4 Corners* program entitled 'Generation Cancer' which examined the cause of an increase in cancer in Australians in their 30s and 40s. There was no commentary provided about the overconsumption of sugar and processed foods and only limited discussion of the underconsumption of vegetables as a potential cause of these cancer increases. Are the sugar industry and the food manufacturers controlling the agenda? Unhealthy food is continually promoted to children who then entrap their parents to do a trip to a takeaway food outlet for dinner. Alternatively, the children are brainwashed by advertising to badger parents to purchase sugary drinks and processed food at the supermarket.

In the past decade, social media has become another fastest growing 'disease' worldwide. It is slowly killing us by depriving us of time, money, exercise and social skills, while generally encouraging us to be unhealthy. Social media can also take credit for a number of psychological problems being experienced by vulnerable social media users.

Sitting at the top of the gravy train is our State and Federal Governments. They don't want to change anything because they are making too much money in taxes on popular but unhealthy foods. They also don't want to upset the co-conspirators as they are heavy hitters.

• • •

In summary, this chapter is designed to be thought-provoking rather than judgemental. The issue is, when does a healthy addiction become an unhealthy addiction and when does it have adverse impacts on our health or longevity? When does an addiction stop giving pleasure and start giving pain? Can the medical profession prescribe exercise and a healthy diet to older people (where appropriate) and less medication? Can we have truthful disclosure about the contents of processed food? Can we spend more money on preventative research?

By pointing out these influences, I don't mean to suggest that people don't need to change – they do. But real change takes willpower, awareness and strong alternative voices. We need to build a culture across all generations that prioritises healthy choices: movement, good nutrition and conscious decision-making. If you take anything from this book – and I hope you take many things – pause and think twice about your daily choices. Your health and wellbeing depend on it.

In the next chapter we will put together the component to create our own blueprint for successful ageing, built on the foundations of positive attitude, exercise, sleep, nutrition, social network supports, avoiding risk factors ... and discover our *ikigai* (our purpose for being).

Before you read on, pause and consider these two questions:

1. **If the evidence is that processed food is killing you, would you be more diligent about what you put in your mouth?**

2. **Would you be prepared to increase your level of exercise and improve your diet if it might increase your health span, reduce your biological age and reduce your level of medication?**

CHAPTER 10: CREATING YOUR OWN BLUEPRINT FOR SUCCESSFUL AGEING

The good news is you don't need to move to Okinawa or Sardinia to experience the benefits of living with a blueprint for successful ageing. In fact, some of these places are very low- or middle-income nations and you would need to sacrifice many of the luxuries we enjoy in Australia. However, you can create your own blueprint for successful ageing and still enjoy the attributes from these locations where you are currently living. The Elders I interviewed identified six components that they attributed to their healthy longevity and successful ageing. The identified components are shown in Figure 10.1, and my plan to make them part of your blueprint for successful ageing is summarised in the following sections.

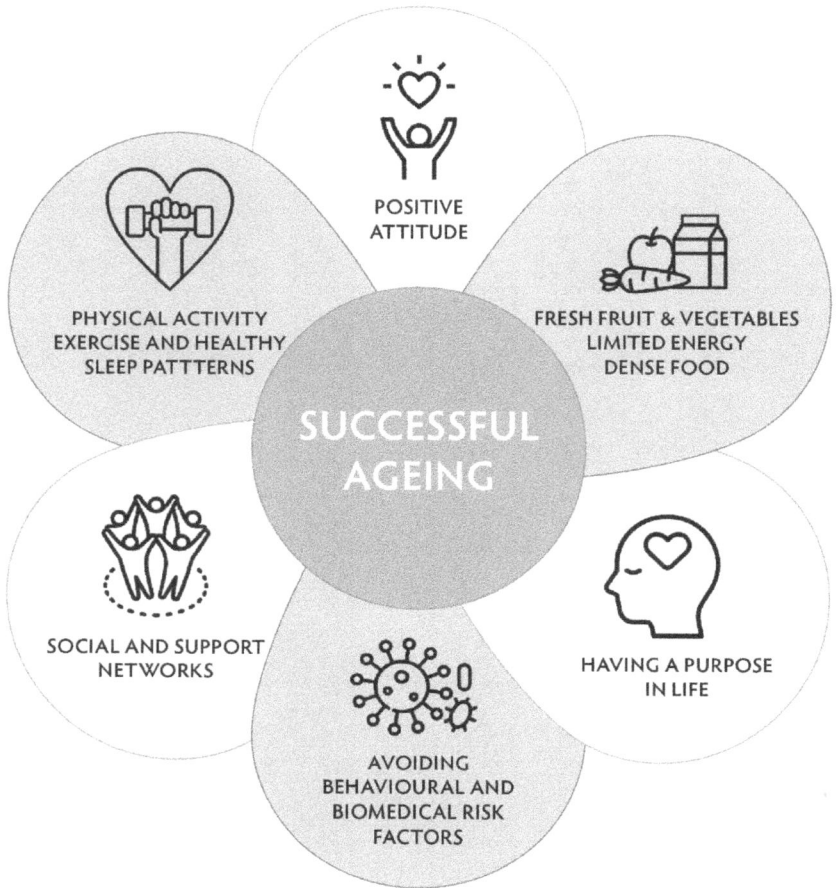

Figure 10.1: Elders' Successful Ageing Components. Source: Interviews with Elders.

Positive attitude

If you have a positive attitude, it provides the catalyst to pursue the successful ageing components in your own environment that will form part of your daily activities. Take pride in your own presentation to the outside world. Some older people are still trendsetters and lead by example for others to follow. If you are clean-shaven and well-groomed, you are more likely to be positive and feel good about yourself. You have got to feel good about yourself if you want others to feel good about you. If you are positive, while still being humble, you will be greeted positively by others. My mother used to say, 'the King is always in the audience'. In other words, you never know who you might meet when you go out.

If we have a positive attitude and are prepared to commit to the successful ageing curve, most of us can create our own blueprint for successful ageing within the environment where we currently live. Older people who are struggling to make ends meet or who are already sick may find it difficult to improve their diet, increase exercise or be more positive. But as we have discussed, even small steps can make a difference. The first step in making a change is to make the decision to make the change. The change may be minor to start with. It might be deciding to go for a walk a few days a week, giving up sugary drinks, or pursuing my 80:20 rule. Remember our previous discussion on habits: when you repeat something a number of times it becomes a habit, which can then become your default reaction.

If you are a naturally positive person, then you will not have difficulty with this starting position. You will likely have the motivation to organise regular exercise and healthy sleep practice: the nucleus for sustaining and rejuvenating the body. However, if you are less positive – we don't use the word 'negative' – you may need some inspiration or role models. I have discussed some of my role models in earlier chapters. The top of my list is Jack LaLanne, who started as a skinny undernourished lad who once wore a back brace, and went on to become the father of gymnasiums. Also, the examples of Jane Fonda, a modern-day role model who recently said she is enjoying life more at 87, than she did when she was in her 20s; Kirk Douglas, who remained active all his life and wrote two bestselling books in his late 90s; George Burns, who was still doing stand-up comedy at 99; and Peter the Centenarian running chef.

Exercise

Exercise is the closest thing to a panacea for successful ageing. It is identified in countless research documents as the most important thing we can do to slow down the ageing process and our biological clock. Hopefully, I have convinced you that your strength and fitness does not need to diminish as you age, if you have the commitment to pursue your desired successful ageing curve.

So, exercise needs to be an integral part of your blueprint for successful ageing. In previous chapters we considered running/walking environments that inspire you. Whether it is a park, the beach, the pool, the golf course – find somewhere you feel good exercising. If you enjoy going there for a walk and meeting a friend, it becomes something you look forward to. I talked earlier about my friend John, who meets a group of people every day and they swim across Bondi Beach and back, about 2km. They then have a coffee and a chat. Similarly, I meet a group two days a week at the pool and we swim a 2km session followed by coffee. Both the swim and the coffee are an enjoyable part of the experience.

We also talked about gym culture, the equipment, the people, and the guidance you might receive from instructors and other members. As I don't wear earpods and don't take my phone, I actually get to talk to others in the gym. It is amazing the friendships you can develop attending a gym regularly and talking to people. I am fortunate to have access to two gymnasiums, both of which I enjoy attending as there is a different group of people at each one. I am on first name terms with almost all, and I enjoy the occasional banter. I don't bother trying to talk to the almost exercisers, who spend more time on their phone than they do exercising, or those who are wired for sound. As discussed, your gym routine is your PEP, which has been developed to achieve your short-, medium- and long-term goals. If gym fees are an issue, there are free outdoor gyms in parks and at beaches. For example, at Bondi Beach there is a very popular outdoor gym that has a variety of equipment.

My earlier recommendation for the pursuit of exercise is at least 60 minutes per day with some vigorous activity included. However, there are many forms of exercise you can pursue. Yoga, which I have attended recently, is incredibly demanding and will build up your strength. Also, Pilates, which I attend once a week, is a great form of exercise. There are many low-cost outdoor exercise opportunities, where instructors offer classes for aerobics, HIIT, running squads and ball games. There are also beach volleyball, tennis and more recently pickleball. Let your environment be your guide and your passion be your advisor. While it is good to try many activities, when you pick one, two or any number of activities that you like, pick and stick. However, ensure that you include strength training in your program.

Don't let your inability to perform an activity prevent you from trying it. I have always had limited natural ability; my only success has come from a stubbornness not to give up. If you're not a good swimmer you will get great physical benefit (as you are less efficient) and you will get immense satisfaction, as your swimming improves. A few years ago, a few Bondi swimmers started a group swim on Fridays and called themselves the Saltys; it has now grown to several hundred. The standard varies immensely, the camaraderie is outstanding, and everyone is made to feel welcome.

Similarly, don't be intimidated by the so-called gym junkies. You will find that most of them will be supportive if you show commitment. You will also develop your mini networks at the beach, pool, gym or park. These groups will become your motivation and a critical part of your blueprint for successful ageing.

With your positive attitude part of your blueprint for successful ageing, introduce exercise into your daily routine for example by leaving the car at home. Walk to the shop, a café for coffee, a friend's place, or if dining locally, walk to and from the restaurant. Walk to the beach to look at the surf or other changing or interesting natural features in your area. Embrace incidental exercise, use the stairs instead of the lift or escalator. Avoid sitting for long periods of time – standing and doing some exercise every half hour is desirable. Learn a package of stretches you can do throughout the day. Use bands, a squeeze ball, a roller and any other aids at home or at work to punctuate your sitting and get your body moving. If you are working, program your exercise before work, lunchtime, after work, or all of the above. Never use the excuse, you don't have time for exercise! It is unacceptable in your blueprint for successful ageing.

Sleep

The understated and most critical element to be able to commit to regular exercise is a good sleep regime. All of the Elders considered that seven to nine hours' good sleep was normal and non-negotiable. As we observed, sleep is the glue that holds mind and body together, that allowed them to pursue exercise and all of the other successful ageing components.

As we observed in Chapter 8, sleep is essential for restoring our bodily functions and deserves separate discussion as a critical part of our blueprint for successful ageing. You will recall we observed that sleep is the sewage system for our brain and the rejuvenator of our body. We noted that there are biological processes occurring during sleep and the brain stores new information and disposes of toxic waste.

Nerve cells communicate and re-organise, which supports brain function. The body repairs cells, restores energy, and releases molecules like hormones and proteins. Sleep allows cells and muscles to repair and regrow. This includes the mitochondria, which is called the powerhouse of the cell, and is present in nearly every cell. Also, the more you tear down the cells and muscles, the stronger they regrow, which in turn pushes back the biological clock.

We previously discussed the reasons why good sleep is essential and they include: energy conservation, cellular reconstruction, brain function and plasticity, emotional wellbeing, weight maintenance, proper insulin function, a healthy strong immune system, heart health, and greater athletic performance. It would seem that there is a compelling argument that our bedroom should be part of our blueprint for successful ageing.

Our behavioural sleep habits are up to the individual – how we prepare for bed, what time we go to bed and get up, what we eat and drink, what we read and what we watch on television. Ideally, going to bed and getting up at the same time is desirable, as well as not eating or drinking two hours before bed, and avoiding coffee and alcohol before bed. These are all good sleep protocols, and they are up to us. However, the bedroom is a sleep zone. As I mentioned, the room needs to be very dark, cool temperature 21-22 degrees Celsius or less (some like it warmer or cooler) and it should be free from distractions: for example, luminous clocks, phones and watches or anything that might keep you from you primary goal of sleep.

Your bed and pillow are considerations that are crucial to establishing your blueprint for successful ageing. The rest, no pun intended, is up to you. It is worth restating the results of the previous study that concluded that men who got adequate sleep lived five years longer, while women who got adequate sleep lived two years longer. The other factor not mentioned is a better quality of life with a good night's sleep.

Nutrition

The nutritional part of your blueprint for successful ageing is also important. Establish connections with the nearest fruit and vegetable shops where there are good sources of plant-based foods, nuts, fruit and vegetables. A good fresh fruit and veg shop is gold. Remember as we age, we need more protein, so you will need to decide whether you eat meat, fish or plants. My preference is some meat, oily fish, plants and plenty of nuts. A good source for fresh fish is important: find a fish shop that goes to the markets regularly; alternatively go direct to the fish markets yourself. Identify the healthy cafés and restaurants and try and avoid the fast food outlets. We have Japanese, Asian and Vietnamese restaurants in close proximity, which we always walk to. Their food is always fresh, wholesome and gluten free. They are an important part of our blueprint for successful ageing.

Reduce your use of the major supermarkets and use them instead of them using you. Remember to shop the periphery and stay away from the so-called healthy (sugary) drinks and foods. Cereal that has over 40% sugar content is not healthy. I recently measured the breakfast cereal – once marketed as 'Iron Man Food' and which is now described on the packet as 'Fuel for Active Bodies' – with my new food packaging app, Yuka. It is marketed at young people and rated 45 out of 100 and is considered to offer poor nutrition. This product is on centre stage in the cereal section. In contrast Gluten Free Weet-Bix scored 90 out of 100 and rated excellent. If goods are largely inaccessible in the supermarket aisles, they are probably good for you. Supermarkets are part of our food network, as most of us don't have access to homegrown vegetables and fruit.

Homegrown and organic vegetables and fruit are awesome, if you have access to them. Increasingly, local areas have farmers' markets once a week, where local and organic vegetables and fruit are available. When we buy the produce direct from the farming community, we are getting fresh fruit and vegetables, helping the farmers survive and avoiding the supermarkets. Getting a fresh supply of nuts and dried fruits is also important. A handful of mixed nuts each day is much better for you than a chocolate bar. Don't just be another customer who walks into a fast food store or supermarket and buys what they are advertising; it is invariably not healthy – do your research!

Think about your weekly meals, plan your dinners, include plenty of vegetables in every meal, and make your kitchen a blueprint for successful ageing. Be guided by the Okinawans' diet and their mantra *hara hachi bu* – serve yourself moderate portions. That means no seconds and no supersizing. Occasionally it is okay to have seconds; if a loved one has prepared a delicious meal, for example, this can be part of your 20%. Try using smaller plates rather than a full-size dinner plate. Also eat no more than three meals a day and don't snack between meals. Remember the 80:20 Rule – eat until you are 80% full. Finally, we all have naughty days, when we eat too much. But try and do the right thing 80% of the time.

Social support networks

The importance of networks cannot be overstated. As we are herd animals, banding together with others is a critical part of our DNA. As you age, these networks include your medical team, GP, cardiologist, sports doctor, physio, massage therapist and other support when necessary. Across the lifespan, they include your friends at the local club, your mates that you went to school or uni with, your church for your spiritual connection and support, and your training buddies at the beach, pool, park, gymnasium, tennis or golf. If one group tells you that you are too old to be involved in an activity, find another group. Also, stay away from the negative people in any group; they will only sap your energy and give you nothing in return. We talked about the Okinawans and their community support group, which is known as the Moai, who are a close group of friends who support each other. If one falls on hard times, the others band together to help. All of your networks have different roles to play and cannot be taken for granted and need to be nurtured. Without connections, older people can become isolated in their homes and lose contact with the outside world. Networks, support groups or your own Moai are an important component of your blueprint for successful ageing.

Avoiding behavioural and biological risk factors

The final component is the epicentre for all of the other components and shows how successful you have been in negotiating life up to this point, by avoiding the life-threatening risk factors. As we discussed, our behavioural risk factors, in a health context, will largely determine how much biological baggage we currently have and carry into our later lives. If you have no biological baggage and you are not taking medication in your 60s, you are in the top 10% of healthy seniors and you deserve a gold star. However, we need to be reminded that a successful ageing blueprint is eternal vigilance; we can never take things for granted and we can always improve.

There are many 50-, 60-, 70- and 80-year-olds who have stopped blaming their parents for their health problems, have thought about healthy longevity, extended their health span, and want to enjoy their last 20 or 30+ years of life. It may be that they are prepared to make a commitment to good health. It is a case of working through each of these components to establish your individual game plan, which will be part of your own personal blueprint for successful ageing. Unless you have a chronic condition or a terminal disease, you can potentially improve your health span, though it does take some serious commitment.

We now have the framework for our blueprint for successful ageing, which we need to cultivate to reap the benefits. We have many advantages over the Blues Zones, with our access to technology, health support and a much higher standard of living. The real problem with civilisation today is that most people are not living in the moment: many are not enjoying our beautiful sunrise and sunsets and are more content on their phones and the various apps that occupy their minds and spirits. Also, they have failed to appreciate how lucky we are to live in this country.

Purpose (*ikigai*)

Ikigai, in its simplest terms, means a purpose for living, or a purpose for getting out of bed in the morning. Having a purpose was a critical component that the Elders identified to give their life meaning. Some Elders were working, while some were caring for others or undertaking voluntary work. A few were studying a language, a musical instrument, a course at university or other passions. I am currently pursuing the trombone and the neighbours in our units regularly go for coffee when I practice. If you don't already have a passion, go out and find one, or a few, that turn you on for the day. It may be helping your local community group. It may be your surf club. It may be your church; find something that gives your day substance and helps you feel that you are giving back and doing something worthwhile. If you have not been involved in helping others before, you will be surprised by how much self-satisfaction and gratitude you will feel in return for your efforts.

• • •

In summary, creating your own blueprint for successful ageing will not be easy. However, the commitment you've shown to reach the (almost) end of this book confirms that you have the positive attitude to achieve your chosen age curve and create your own blueprint for successful ageing.

As I keep saying, your chronological age is irrelevant: it is your biological age which matters, and you can lower your biological age. Remember, *if you think you can, or if you think you can't, you are probably right!*

In the last chapter I will deliver some final thoughts on my journey, share the eight important lessons I have learnt during my lifetime, and offer you my closing pitch to change your life. There will then be a few after thoughts following our visit to Okinawa and Japan.

Before you read on, pause and consider these two questions:

1. **Do you have a positive attitude towards life generally? Can you name three things that you are grateful for?**

2. **What is your *ikigai* – your purpose for living? If you don't have one, give it some thought over the next 24 hours. (Chances are your *ikigai* is found at the intersection of what you love most, what you are good at, and the thing that most enriches your days, even without the need for payment.)**

CHAPTER 11: FINAL THOUGHTS

I am honoured that I have been able to share some of my experiences with you and that you have managed to make it through to my concluding chapter. My hope is that this book will inspire and encourage you to think about what you can do to build yourself a better future. Although the past 80 years have not been without their challenges, I am incredibly fortunate to have been able to continue to reside in Bondi, to pursue my chosen professional life, to remain married to an amazing woman for 54 years and to retain a level of fitness where I can still undertake my favourite activities.

When I first joined the surf club in 1964, I would never have thought that I would still be competing, at the NSW and Australian Surf Life Saving Championships, 60 years down the track in 2025. It was never my intention to be the oldest competitor in the North Bondi club to win a gold medal at those championships; however, having achieved that unlikely recognition, I do feel incredibly proud.

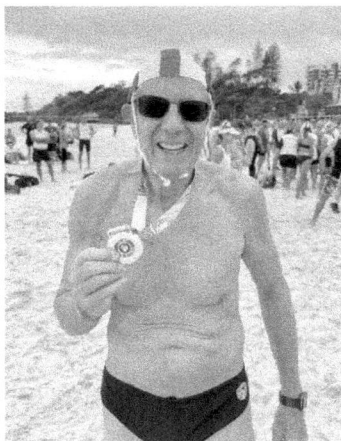

The author pictured after his gold medal winning race in the over 75 years, 1km soft sand race, at the Australian Masters Championships, at Kirra in 2025.

In the past 10 years, I have experienced an injury to each shoulder, which had some serious repercussions. It would have been easy to give up competition or indeed give up exercise altogether. When I tore the first supraspinatus tendon approximately six years ago trying to paddle through a largish wave at Bondi, and received my diagnosis, I thought my paddling days were over. I'm also reminded of my surgeon's quip, that a person my age, then 74, normally tears this tendon falling out of bed, rather than paddling a surf ski. Little did I realise that it would be 12 months rehab and another four lots of surgery, including the same injury to the other shoulder and an ablation, just to mention a few, that I would experience in the next six years. I am fortunate to be a typical Capricorn and burdened with those Capricorn traits, where the goat is always climbing the mountain and doesn't know when to give up.

There have certainly been many occasions when life seemed too difficult, and I could have gone in a different direction. The loss of our son Ryan is the singular most painful event of my life. Exercise was my saviour and thank God, my marriage endured. The loss of Ryan did convince me that I should not waste my life and that I also needed to be living life for both of us.

Living with and caring for my old Mum was another salutary experience, which helped me to appreciate how healthy ageing is a potential bonus that most Australians don't grasp by the throat. We need to work hard in order to enjoy the last 10 or 20 years of life. The professional work I did with aged care providers and facilities convinced me that taking it easy and sitting around in the twilight of life is not the blueprint for successful ageing.

While I thought completing the four-day ski paddling marathon from Forster to Bondi was the most difficult thing I would ever undertake, it paled into insignificance with the 10-year journey for my PhD on ageing. To be told after nine years I didn't have the expertise for the topic I was pursuing was amazingly stressful. One can either look at these events and feel sorry for oneself or accept the challenge. Challenges are character-building; they define who you are and what you will be in later years. Perhaps these events have been responsible for my obsessive-compulsive behaviour, which I would like to think will stand by me for my next 20 years.

I need to confess, I cannot guarantee you that my strategy, paradigm and blueprint for successful ageing is correct or that my philosophy on exercise is irrefutable. I can say that it is based on my lifetime of experience, both personal and the observations of others, that I have carefully documented. My research has also considered the relevant data, the research relating to exercise and the nutritional guidelines that are readily available for everyone, yet so many in our population seem to ignore (and are becoming progressively unhealthy in the process). As people age and become immobile or bedridden, it is easy for doctors to say, 'This is part of the ageing process'. As I have said and firmly believe, decline, disability, decrepitude, disease and dependency are not inevitable. I have used myself as a test dummy for the different types of exercise as I have aged, to determine what was best for me, at ages 50, 60, 70 and now 80 and I have documented those findings. I also test drove the various diets, discussed earlier, and recorded what worked and what didn't. Remember, when we put food in our mouth, we are either feeding disease or fighting it. Sadly, only a few members of the population take the time to work out what exercise they should be doing, and which foods are best for them. Our objective is to extend our health span to equal our lifespan.

As I have said throughout this book, ageing is not the problem or a disease, the disease is being sedentary, and this is now recognised by the WHO. We are also being poisoned by much of the food we consume. Our bodies are designed to move, and they function more efficiently when we move them regularly and vigorously. As we age, our strength, muscle mass and wellbeing will decline if we don't look after where we live, our bodies. One of my mantras that I keep repeating is, 'you have got to look after your body; it is the only place you have to live'. In my paradigm, chronological age is just a number, and we need to work on lowering our biological age. My philosophy is exercise is the closest thing to a panacea for successful ageing. The previously mentioned study of one million people supports my philosophy. Any exercise is good, more is better, and vigorous is best. In other words, the more we undertake programmed exercise, the healthier we age.

Jack LaLanne's mantra continues to inspire me: 'Exercise is King. Nutrition is Queen. Put them together, and you have a Kingdom.' Or, in our case, you have your blueprint, at least the beginning of it!

The many components for looking after the body include nutrition and sleep. It really is most unfortunate that we are misled by food manufacturers, supermarkets and the media to consume food that is killing us. It is even more unfortunate that food manufacturers are allowed to put salt, sugar and various additives into food that are potentially carcinogenic. We need to take control of our own ageing. Most of our population have every opportunity to exercise regularly, eat healthy, drink plenty of water, get a good night's sleep, and ensure they satisfy their social, intellectual, community and spiritual needs. Yet many of us choose to disregard healthy ageing guidelines.

If you have been convinced to pursue one of my top two ageing curves, then you have probably realised you'll need to make some significant lifestyle changes. Please don't look at these changes as a sacrifice: consider them as being an investment in the future and you will look forward to improved lifestyle and quality of life in the coming decades. If you feel you are stuck on the third or typical ageing curve, try and make just a few improvements to your lifestyle; you may be surprised how much better you feel. As James Clear popularised in his book *Atomic Habits*, by applying the 1% rule, even a 1% daily cumulative improvement can bring about major changes.

There is much talk about longevity and living forever and a lot of people forget to live for the now. The main message I would like to convey is to enjoy every moment of every day as you do not know how many days you have left on this amazing planet. If you can enjoy the moment and be positive about ageing, longevity will take care of itself.

Life's lessons

The final part of this chapter includes the lessons I have learnt during my lifetime and my closing pitch to change your life.

Lesson 1 – *Create your own Blueprint for Successful Ageing*

The most important lesson I have learnt is the benefit of creating your own blueprint for successful ageing. Your blueprint can be in one location, or like my circumstances, spread to several locations. For exercise I am fortunate to have the beach in close proximity, where I use the water and the sand for various activities; coastline and parks for walking; two gymnasiums; and a nearby golf course. I also enjoy skiing in Thredbo and Perisher in Australia, and overseas where possible. Also, my stand-up desk helps me get incidental exercise, while I am working at the computer. My outdoor and indoor activities offer me a series of social networks, which I enjoy immensely, and receive valuable friendship and stimulation. My wife and I have largely a plant-based diet, with fish and occasionally meat, and we mainly eat at home. When we go out to restaurants, it's always a healthy selection and we avoid deep fried and refined foods. Our sleep habits are healthy and regularised, and we both have a purpose in life. We apply the 80:20 Rule, and we avoid behavioural and biomedical risk factors.

Creating your own blueprint for successful ageing is bringing healthy ageing components into your life, rather than moving to Okinawa or Sardinia, where these components may or may not exist.

Lesson 2 – *Mentoring is a great gift*

Mentoring and passing on thoughtful and constructive advice to younger or less-experienced people is one of the most satisfying things you can do, and one of the greatest gifts you can receive.

I am fortunate to have been mentored several times during my life. When I first joined the surf club; when I started life as an engineering surveyor then town planner; through my university years and then by my supervisors completing my PhD. In return, I have endeavoured to pass forward or give back my experiences to others in those same forums. I've always tried to provide advice to anyone who is requesting any form of guidance. In the surf club I have been a competitor, trainer, coach, mentor, sponsor and I am currently the Patron. In my planning practice I always aimed to encourage and support young planners, and I still stay in touch with a few of my previous employees. I also endeavour to make presentations and advise on healthy ageing to anyone who is interested. Currently, I offer advice to a number of friends when they ask for it. It is interesting how the problems that I have had to deal with over the years keep reoccurring for others. It is always a pleasure to be able to share my experiences and to caution them not to make the same mistakes that I made.

Lesson 3 – Spending time with elite athletes and gifted people

Training with elite athletes makes you fitter, faster and stronger, and provides an exceptional opportunity to learn and improve. Also, working with or spending time with people who are cleverer than you, or have a different skill set, helps to lift you up to their level or learn new things.

While this lesson applies primarily to exercise, it is equally relevant for life. Attending conferences where elite speakers can inspire and inform is important for self-development. I recall attending an Anthony Robbins weekend and walking on hot coals in Darling Harbour at 11pm. He convinced me of the importance of a positive attitude, which was borne out by the Elders in our interviews. In my planning practice, I always aimed to employ the smartest and hardest-working employees I could find. I encouraged and supported young intelligent staff members with the right attitude as they would pay dividends in the long run and in turn get the most benefit from my advice.

Lesson 4 – *Prepare your personal exercise program (PEP) to meet your short-, medium- and long-term goals*

After deciding on your long-term goal(s), you can decide on the short- and medium-term goals that will get you there. The next step is developing a PEP, perhaps with a trainer, to ensure maximum benefit in the time available. Remember your PEP is designed to help you achieve your long-term goal(s). Exercise is a priority so decide when it best fits into your day and lock it in.

Time is a precious commodity, and we need to use it as efficiently and effectively as possible. Accordingly, your PEP can be an essential part of your daily life and be the centrepiece when organising your daily activities.

Lesson 5 – *Test your limits and commit*

You don't know your limits until you are truly tested. Another of my philosophies is that, 'if you are not living life on the edge, you are taking up too much space!' However, you need to accept that if you live life on the edge, you will occasionally fall off. In other words, you need to be continually challenging yourself, whether it is exercise, study or working to achieve your long-term goals. Life needs to be a process of organised challenges. Life will provide its own challenges that are totally unprogrammed. If you are used to meeting challenges, the unprogrammed ones will be more readily dealt with. As the Ancient Greeks said, 'knowing thyself is the beginning of wisdom.' Keep testing and committing until it becomes a habit. Whether it is exercise, what we eat, how we sleep, or the way we connect, we improve when we test our limits, and those limits become habits. We are what we repeatedly do.

Lesson 6 – Preparation is key to gaining results

Benjamin Franklin is credited with saying: 'If you fail to plan, you are planning to fail.' I've always believed that preparation is the key to success. Whether it is preparing for an event, an exam, a presentation to a board or an audience, you're only as good as your preparation. When you properly prepare, you are aware of any shortcomings, and you resolve them before there is a drama. I can recall occasions when I was not properly prepared for a presentation or an event, and it was a disaster. When you are properly prepared you are confident that you will perform well on the stage or on the sporting field.

Lesson 7 – Engage in a variety of exercises, at any age

The Elders proved we can pursue a variety of exercises at any age, and it can be enjoyable and satisfying while being good for our physical and mental needs. I've enjoyed a variety of exercises which vary with the seasons, and I am fortunate enough to be able to pursue most activities I enjoy. I can run, swim, paddle a surf ski, go to the gym, play golf, go skiing, play pickleball and play trombone (badly). I have been told not to play tennis, which I previously enjoyed, as I have another minor tear in the supraspinatus tendon. I'm also restricted from chin-ups, dips, and a few other exercises I used to enjoy in the gym. However, this is a small price to pay.

In my opinion, your PEP should include at least two strength and two cardio routines per week. Also, golf is fine, Pilates is good, running is great, and swimming is excellent. Additionally, don't forget the abs, stretching and balance.

Lesson 8 – Pursue aerobic and strengthening exercise for 60 minutes per day, 6 days a week

I cannot overstate the importance of pursuing weights in a gym at least twice a week, preferably three times. My PEP has a minimum of two strength exercise routines a week. At my age, muscle mass and strength are quickly lost without doing weights. Bands and pulleys are good, but it is difficult to get the loading required to build or maintain muscle. In contrast, aerobic exercise can be achieved in a variety of ways including running (including on the soft sand), swimming, rowing, ski paddling, HIIT, and a number of gym machines. An additional bonus from soft sand running is a loss of body fat, as well as being an excellent form of aerobic exercise.

My closing pitch

As I conclude this book, it is important that I summarise the potential qualitative and quantitative benefits from creating your own blueprint for successful ageing and pursuing a successful ageing curve. The 10 benefits from moving onto this curve, which can transform your life, are:

- The likelihood of an improved quality of life and general wellbeing.
- The potential to be active, vital and connected with people, for the whole of life.
- An extension of health span to almost equal your lifespan.
- Lifespan bonus years: positive attitude 7.5, correct weight 10, sleep 5 (males), 2 (females).
- Increased muscle mass, strength, flexibility and balance, with a strong metabolism.
- A reduced chance of being diagnosed with cancer, or heart and brain-related diseases.
- Avoidance or deferment of sarcopenia, and reduced risk of falls.
- The potential to reduce medication or avoid it altogether.
- Improved pattern and quality of sleep; and
- The likelihood of less or no time spent in the disability zone.

In my 80th year I achieved my two short-term goals, which gave me the leg strength to achieve my two medium-term goals of powder skiing and running on soft sand. My long-term goal was running in the soft sand race at the Aussie Championships, and I prepared my PEP for that challenge, and secondly, completing this book and making my website more interactive. These long-term goals are works in progress. Thirdly, I have recently completed my tour of Okinawa and Japan, and I have discussed the findings previously and in my Afterword.

As I look at life beyond 80, I'm confident I've developed an approach that will support me in subsequent years. I may need to ease back a tad on my personal challenges. My research, interviews, lifestyle and life experience observing others have taught me many lessons. I keep myself accountable as I enact my own lifestyle and fitness changes, and I believe sharing these will open the door for those of you who are either struggling with a setback or who simply want to live better. Although we might plan for a healthy long life, we don't know what life has in store for us around the corner. Accordingly, it is important to live in the present and enjoy the moment!

My current *ikigai* is to provide as many people as possible with the information to assist them to develop their own blueprint for successful ageing!

I wish you well in your journey as you age and hope you feel better equipped to create changes that will make a fantastic difference. Hopefully, this book has convinced you that you are never too young or too old to embrace the challenge of successful ageing. I look forward to continuing to learn and age successfully as I commence my 90th decade, and I wish you well on your journey.

Remember, chronological age is just a number, it is your biological age which is important, and you can control your biological age!

AFTERWORD

Before finishing this book, Vicki and I travelled to Okinawa – one of the original Blue Zones – to see if spending extended time there might be a practical option for healthy longevity. Could living there help me live longer and better? Could it be an example others might follow?

It quickly became clear that, in reality, relocating there or spending extended time there – especially for someone in their later years – is simply not realistic. Few would want to, and fewer still have the means. You would be far from friends and family, from a familiar health system, from a lifetime of social ties – and without these, the community bond that gives Blue Zones their power simply isn't there for you.

The trip got off to an unfortunate start. When we arrived at Naha Airport, the car rental company refused to hire to drivers over 70 – ironic in a region celebrated for its centenarians. We did find another company which was not age discriminatory, but the message was clear: even in the Blue Zones, being a long-lived person can be a disadvantage.

My wife and I drove to the northernmost tip of Okinawa and travelled both on the eastern and western side of the island down to, and past, Naha – a city of around 300,000 inhabitants, a size analogous to Newcastle in NSW. We also visited a pleasant small village known as Ogimi, featured in Dan Buettner's *The Blue Zone* book and referred to in Drs Bradley and Craig Willcox and Makoto Suzuki's book *The Okinawa Program*. The village of Ogimi is spread out and is located south of the national park. The sign at the entry to the village states: *At 70 you are but a child, at 80 you are merely a youth, and at 90 if the ancestors invite you into heaven, ask them to wait until you are 100 … then you might consider it.*

The first thing I observed was the lush vegetation that is everywhere, particularly along the roads we travelled. I use the word lush rather than sub-tropical, which is what I was expecting. I had this image in my mind of rows and rows of palm trees. Also along the roadside are clusters of tombs, where the Okinawans bury their families – a striking reminder of how Okinawans honour their ancestors. This custom started many years ago, when vacant strips or parcels of land, close to transport, were seconded by locals, and tombs were constructed that can hold the whole family. Okinawans regularly visit these sites, or roadside cemeteries, to pay their respects to family who have passed.

But the villages themselves, like Ogimi, the so-called longevity capital, were far quieter than I expected. The reality is that the younger generations have left for work in the cities, leaving many houses vacant or falling into disrepair. It was over 35 degrees Celsius most days, which partly explained the empty streets, but the sense of decline was unmistakable.

I had imagined charming traditional Japanese houses – instead, we found concrete or timber dwellings, small, weathered, often lacking any clear property boundaries, some looking untouched since World War II. It made sense why these communities have historically been so tight-knit – they lived practically in each other's front yards. But now, with the young gone, many neighbourhoods feel hollowed out.

At the same time, we found moments that revealed why this culture still produces such long-lived people. The food was simple, fresh and mostly unprocessed. Breakfasts of tofu, rice and salad were worlds apart from the sugary cereals so many Australians eat – I lost two kilograms without trying. Smaller plates, chopsticks, and the mindful practice of eating only until 80 per cent full – these small habits shape health in ways we can adopt anywhere.

We stayed in beachside hotels at Okuma Beach and Cape Zanpa. The hospitality was exceptional, the food honest and generous. Yet it was striking how hard it was to find traditional Japanese accommodation in Okinawa – we had to wait for Kyoto for that.

The presence of the US military – a remnant of WWII – is still visible in Okinawa. There are large bases, fast food chains, vending machines for Coca-Cola everywhere you look. In some places, it was easier to find a Big Mac than a tofu salad. Commercial tourism has taken hold, too – parts of the coastline are dotted with luxury resorts for well-heeled travellers.

One thing that stayed with me was the lack of conversation. Few people were out and about, and we found it hard to connect – no Moai or natural support network we could tap into, only polite but brief exchanges.

After Okinawa, we flew to Hiroshima – confronting and humbling in its own way. Visiting the museum and the epicentre of where the atomic bomb was dropped on August 6, 1945 reminded us how recent history's horrors can shape a people's humility and calmness in the face of hardship. Out of a total population of 255,000 in Hiroshima, 66,000 were killed and 69,000 injured (a total of 135,000). Many more died in the next 12 months. They say that people are still dying today, from the effects of the radiation. It was confronting, to say the least.

In Kyoto, we finally saw the traditional Japanese housing I had expected to find in Okinawa: narrow streets, small parcels of land, and historic Japanese architecture that has stood the test of time. Early in the mornings we went walking around the historic village where our hotel was located. These areas had signs which, when translated, read 'silver zone', reflecting that many long-lived people lived in this location. The narrow streets, the absence of parking for larger cars, and the way people made use of every bit of space reminded me of similar issues we face in the inner suburbs of Sydney. One morning, I saw a senior person doing Tai Chi – so focused he didn't even notice me trying to speak with him – so I settled for a photograph instead.

Our next stop was Tokyo. The city's streetscape revealed another lesson – thoughtful urban design that respects the tactile strips for the vision-impaired, audible bird calls at crossings for the blind, and beautifully maintained parks where people of all ages gather to move, stretch and connect.

These places reminded me that the heart of any Blue Zone isn't just its food or scenery – it's the social fabric, the respect for Elders, the built environments that foster connection. These are things you cannot parachute into in old age – you have to build them over a lifetime or adopt their lessons where you already live.

On the flight home, I knew with certainty that moving to Okinawa or any other place in the so-called Blue Zones – for me or for any other older Australian – makes no sense. There is too much you leave behind: family, friends, community, a health system, the ties that bind you to your own place. The truth is, there is little to be gained by physically relocating – but everything to be gained by learning.

If there was one standout of our time in Japan, it would be respect. Bowing when greeting and saying goodbye is infectious and humbling. The Japanese try hard to leave people feeling better after they have greeted them. Also, closeness of family, Moai and friends, and endearing treatment of family even in death, and revering long-lived people.

What we can bring back is the best of what Okinawan and Japanese cultures offer: the mindful eating, the humility and politeness, the built form that supports healthy movement and connection, the way families and neighbours look out for each other, and the daily rituals that remind people they matter.

These are the elements we can weave into our lives, our families, our neighbourhoods – no matter where we live. That is the real path to ageing well. The secret is not in moving somewhere new, but in letting what you learn shape the way you live now.

I'm glad we went, and I was glad to come home again – to my own Moai, at North Bondi, the place I have lived all my life. It put the Blue Zones into perspective and reminded me that the real journey is not about geography – it's about living with purpose, respect and connection, wherever you call home. You don't need to move across the world to do it – you can build your own version of a Blue Zone right where you are. I call it a blueprint for successful ageing.

FURTHER READING

Attia, P. & Gifford B. (2023). *Outlive: The science and art of longevity.* Vermilion.

Bernard, N. (2013). *Power foods for the brain.* Hachette.

Bortz, W. (1991). *We live too short and die too long.* Bantam Books.

Brewer, S. & Kellow, J. (2018). *Eat better, live longer: Understand what your body needs to stay healthy.* Penguin.

Buettner, D. (2008). *The Blue Zone: Lessons for living longer from the people who've lived the longest.* National Geographic.

Campbell, T. C. & Campbell, T. M. (2016). *The China Study: The most comprehensive study of nutrition ever conducted and the startling implications for diet, weight loss and long-term health.* BenBella Books.

Clear, J. (2018). *Atomic habits.* Penguin.

Crowley, C., & Lodge, H. S. (2004). *Younger next year: A guide to living like 50 until you're 80 and beyond.* Workman Publishing.

D'Adamo, P. (1998). *The eat right diet: A simple guide to eating right.* Century.

Di Lorenzo, S. (2024). *My Mediterranean life: Recipes and stories.* Simon & Schuster.

Evans, W., Rosenberg, I. H. & Thompson, J. (1991). *Biomarkers: The 10 determinants of Ageing you can control.* Simon & Schuster.

Ferguson, M. (2009). *The aquarian conspiracy: Personal and social transformation in the 1980s.* Tarcher.

Frankl, V. (2011). *Man's search for meaning.* Random House.

Garcia, H. & Miralles, F. (2017). *Ikigai: The Japanese secret to a long and happy life.* Hutchinson Publishing.

Gillespie, D. (2017). *Sweet poison: Why sugar is making us fat.* Penguin.

Harari, Y. N. (2015). *Sapiens: A brief history of humankind.* Vintage Arrow.

Heidrich, R. (2005). *Senior fitness: The diet and exercise program for maximum health and longevity.* Lantern Books.

Izzo, J. (2018). *The five secrets you must discover before you die.* Penguin.

Key, S. (2007). *The back sufferers' bible.* Allen & Unwin.

Lustig, R. (2021). *Metabolical: The truth about processed food and how it poisons people and the planet.* Yellow Kite.

McKeith, G. (2006), *You are what you eat.* Penguin.

Moseley, M. & Spencer, M. (2014). *The fast diet: The simple secret of intermittent fasting.* Short Books.

Paffenbarger, R. & Olsen, E. (1996). *LifeFit.* Human Kinetics Publishers.

Ratey, J. & Hagerman, E. (2008). *Spark: The revolutionary new science of exercise and the brain.* Little Brown.

Robbins, J. (2006). *Healthy at 100: How to extend your life and stay fit!* Hodder & Stoughton.

Root, L. & Kiernan, T. (1985). *Oh, my aching back.* Penguin.

Rowe, J. W. & Kahn, R. L. (1998). *Successful aging.* Pantheon Books.

Servan-Schreiber, D. (2010). *AntiCancer: A new way of life.* Penguin.

Willcox, J., Willcox, C., & Makoto Suzuki. (2002). *The Okinawa Program: How the world's longest-lived people achieve everlasting health – and how you can too.* Harmony.

www.ingramcontent.com/pod-product-compliance
Ingram Content Group Australia Pty Ltd
76 Discovery Rd, Dandenong South VIC 3175, AU
AUHW011203281125
420181AU00006B/8